FAST FORWARD

FAST FORWARD

THE AUTOBIOGRAPHY

The hard road to football success

ANDREW COLE

With Leo Moynihan

HODDER &
STOUGHTON

First published in Great Britain in 2020 by Hodder & Stoughton
An Hachette UK company

1

Copyright © Andrew Cole 2020

A CIP catalogue record for this title is available from the British Library

Hardback ISBN 9781529304954
Trade Paperback ISBN 9781529304961
eBook ISBN 9781529304978

Typeset in Sabon by Palimpsest Book Production Ltd, Falkirk, Stirlingshire

Printed and bound in Great Britain by Clays Ltd, Elcograf S.p.A.

Hodder & Stoughton policy is to use papers that are natural, renewable
and recyclable products and made from wood grown in sustainable forests.
The logging and manufacturing processes are expected to conform to the
environmental regulations of the country of origin.

Hodder & Stoughton Ltd
Carmelite House
50 Victoria Embankment
London EC4Y 0DZ

www.hodder.co.uk

CONTENTS

*For my family. My grandparents, my parents
and my two beautiful children, Devante and Faith.
Without them, nothing was possible.*

FOREWORD

The reason for signing Andy Cole was our own recent success, which had resulted in our opponents changing their tactics. They started defending deeper and I felt we needed someone with an electricity in and around the penalty box. That man was Andy Cole, and it changed our attacking dramatically.

Over the five and a half years he was with us, Andy improved his overall game to a very high standard but, on top of that, just look at his goal record – 231 starts, 121 goals.

He also made forty-four substitute appearances, which brought out the disapproval in Andy's demeanour. He did not like being left out and would walk by me without saying a word, despite my call of 'Morning, Andy!' This usually lasted until the Thursday prior to a game, when I would start to get a 'Morning, boss!' in response.

He is an independent young man, which is based on his pride and his faith in himself, and he has a great strength of character. I must also mention that he was always an immaculate, smart dresser!

His overall contribution at United is something I will always be thankful for and, in my book, he deservedly joins the pantheon of our great players.

Sir Alex Ferguson

1
SHOW US YOUR MEDALS (AND PILLS)

I'm not sure whether life prepared me for football, or football prepared me for life. I'd never be arrogant enough to say I cracked either, but I have given them a good go. In both I have experienced glory and despair. Both have asked me to show my strengths, both have tested my weaknesses.

In football, I have played for the biggest of clubs, scored 187 Premier League goals (only Alan Shearer and Wayne Rooney have more), won trophies, including five Premier League titles and a Champions League, taken adulation and suffered humiliation. Defeats and triumphs in, fortunately, unequal measure.

In life, I have known joy, fathered the most beautiful and loving of children, been part of the most supportive family, taken that support through a serious illness and faced both my demons and my own mortality, learning the hard way that tomorrow can simply be the most satisfying of targets.

Being in the public eye, you do have to deal with the perceptions of others, but the goldfish bowl of supposed fame was never for me. I grew up with a football in my hands and the game in my heart, desperate to play it at the highest level, but that love and desire for football was confined to the markings of the pitch on which I played. Celebrity and notoriety were never driving forces, but I learnt quickly that they come with the territory. I can look back now and say I didn't handle that side of things well, but I was only being myself. Because I hadn't sought it out, I drew away from it, and with that people started to make up their minds about me.

To the press and to the public, I became this supposed loner, dismissive of others, aloof. That last one makes me think. Aloof? For so long, I did tend to deal with things internally, coping with it all my way, and when I now look back at two seminal moments in my career and my life, in each one I was alone.

The first incident was in Barcelona, the Nou Camp. A balmy May night in 1999. On the face of it, I was far from alone. There were 60,000 Manchester United fans with me. United had just beaten Bayern Munich after the craziest end to any game I was ever involved in and won the Champions League, to go with the Premier League title and the FA Cup.

Raw emotion. To win it with two late goals, to win

the Treble in such a dramatic way, spoke volumes for the team and a club ethos that never says, 'Enough.' Piles of players, hugs with staff, tears, joy and song. But I wanted to be alone, just for a few minutes, and so I took myself into an empty spot on the pitch. I looked into a sea of punters. I could see the pure joy in their eyes, expressions that make what we do so special.

I knew that what we had just done had been the most momentous of group efforts. Players, those fans, an army of staff – we had all pulled together and made history. As I stood alone, though, I allowed my mind to drift and think of the people who weren't there. My mum and my dad, my brother, sisters; a family who had supported me, who had made sure that I got to games, that I had football boots. The lads, older and younger than me, who shared park pitches with me as a boy, playing from morning until night during our long, hot summers. They were all in my mind.

I thought of my grandad, Vincent. Vincent had died a couple of years before, a loss that had saddened me more than I could communicate at the time, and as I looked up at the supporters starting a party that would go on for days, I thought of this wonderful man from Jamaica who had so wanted me to play this strange English game. He didn't know much about football, but he knew I could play and never stopped encouraging me to do so. He had missed my most memorable achievement, but as

I stood alone under that Iberian sky, he was with me and I smiled.

Fast-forward almost twenty years and once again I was alone. This time in my bedroom at home. I had come from hospital, where, because of renal failure, I had had a kidney transplant. In front of me were the pills I now had to take, many of them for the rest of my life. I'd tipped out a big bag of medication and the twenty-odd boxes lay spread across the carpet. This was it. This was my new reality.

I began to cry. I was shaking. The emotion was one thing, but my high dosage of everything from antifungal meds to aspirin for thinning my blood had me trembling. I dropped to the floor. This was not for me. I was not having it. There I was, quitting in the room. Lying on a sea of pills, ready to drown.

What I didn't know then was that I was mourning a former life. A life of athleticism, achievement and glory. For twenty years, I had been a professional footballer. I had shown great promise as a kid, been recognised at every level internationally, fought against any doubters that came my way, scored goals and won trophies. The pinnacle was that night in Barcelona and the days that followed.

Immediately after the game, the celebrations went

straight into full swing. You won't see me in many photos after the game, though, because that quiet contemplation I mentioned continued. I talked to team-mates, a grin across my face. I talked to staff, and the gaffer, with knowing looks just as meaningful as the biggest of bear hugs.

But when we returned to Manchester and I saw a river of red awaiting us, I knew that this was the time. I was going to be front and centre. This was *the* moment. Dwight Yorke (my great mate, who is never shy of the limelight) was with me. Teddy Sheringham (my not so great mate) was with me. No time for grudges. This team had achieved something and no one had ever seen Manchester like it.

When you are up on a bus like that, slowly moving through a mass of people, you look closely and you see not just a joyous crowd, but individuals. It's those expressions etched on face after face that bring home what you have achieved. Yes, we footballers want to be successful, but I have always wanted to go out on a Saturday and score goals, knowing that you are making individual lives a little bit happier.

Throughout the twenty years since Manchester United won that Treble, I haven't stopped meeting people wanting to take me back there. I'm not one to look backwards, but how can we not when it comes to the mad events of 1999? What always gets me is just how invested those punters are in what we were doing. 'That night in Barcelona changed my life, for ever,' they'll say, or, 'I was in Turin that night we beat Juventus and I've never been prouder of us.'

Us. It's the right word. When you achieve so much at a club like Manchester United it's all about that collective, and when I take a rare moment to look back on my career at all the clubs I was at, I am obviously proud, but also so grateful to so many people who worked alongside me.

Perhaps that's what has made my illness so hard to take. For so long, my battle with my medication and their side effects was far from a team game. It was me against my pills, and for long periods I was two goals down with only minutes to go.

I was low. So low. Thoughts of quitting were never far away, and the closer they got, the more withdrawn I became at home. This was me coping alone, trying to convince myself that I didn't need medication, that I wasn't even that ill; this was me coping my way, as I had so many times in my career, but little did I know that I was doing myself even more harm.

When you have an organ transplant, and it is successful, you are greeted with smiles. That's that done. You're cured. But a transplant is just the start. Yes, it gives you a chance – and I will never be able to thank my nephew Alexander enough for giving up his kidney to give me that chance – but the struggle starts right away, and when I faced those first stages of a new life, I went lower than I had ever been.

Medically, the support was phenomenal. Continued tests, pills, brilliant consultants checking you out regularly. The thing is, those check-outs stretch only to the physical. Mentally, there is no support. I have never been one to ask for help, and so none came forth. I was showing no signs of the mental hardship I was feeling as I was keeping it all inside, typically storing it, compressing it, ignoring it, not realising it could blow.

Self-doubts were constant. I wasn't sure I could cope with this new life. I hadn't chosen it, I was angry with it. Why me, for God's sake? All self-indulgent stuff, but I wasn't prepared for the mental side of things. My marriage wasn't coping with the illness either. I wanted support; my wife, Shirley, wanted to manage. That's how I saw things.

Lower and lower I went. More distant. More arguments. There were times in those first months after my 2017 transplant that I wondered about ending it. I felt the pills were ending me, so why not just give them a helping hand? There were too many battles and I felt I was losing them all.

*

One battle I wasn't even aware I was having was between my body and my mind. Since falling ill in 2015, my mind had rejected my illness.

'You have kidney failure, Mr Cole.'

'OK, whatever, it'll pass. Give me some pills.'

'The medication isn't working, Mr Cole. We need to find a donor.'

'Nah, no need for that, the pills will work.'

And on it went. So much so that immediately after my transplant, I started to suffer seizures. Not that I believed it. Shirley would notice them while I was sleeping. *Don't be silly.* Then one day in hospital, my nephew was with me as I slept. I woke up to find him panicking, saying I had been having a seizure. A specialist finally diagnosed non-epileptic disorder. Basically, it was the power of the mind. I had kept so much in, tried for years to convince myself that I was well, that my mind was sending the wrong information to my body and, snap, my body couldn't cope.

As a boy and a young footballer, I had wanted to do things my way. When I was only fourteen, *The Times* did a small article on me. Arsenal had signed me and I was among the sixteen best players of my age selected to go to the FA National School at Lilleshall in Shropshire. The journalist wrote about my promise, before saying, 'Andrew Cole could go all the way . . . if he doesn't self-destruct.'

He must have had a tip-off. That was me. Impulsive. I'd act now and think later. Sure, on a football pitch, that fearless trait might be beneficial, but there are times in life when your mind needs to step back and do the right thing. Now, with a serious illness facing me for the rest of my days, this was that time.

I remember one day I was really low and my mum could see that I was close to giving up. 'Andrew,' she said in a way that, however old you are, makes a son take notice, 'you are not a quitter, you never have been and it isn't starting now.' Mum, and my immediate family, knew all about my character. They knew I would always fight my corner, often with disastrous consequences, but there and then she wanted to see that side of me again. It was time to listen to Mum.

At the end of 2017, my marriage was over. With hindsight, it had been for a very long time, but since September 2018, I have lived alone. Not a problem, but it has made me think. When my twenty-seven-year relationship with Shirley came to an end, it was clear I was struggling to cope. My mum's words were in my head, but I needed more. The seizures, the depression: it was obvious that my kidney was not the only thing that needed treatment.

Like so many men, I was reluctant, but I began to

have counselling, and it was the best thing I have ever done. I had to let things go. Having been so ill, I had foolishly felt that, like the attentions of a brutish centre-half, I could simply beat it with a will to win. No chance. The illness was like a pressure cooker and the lid was about to come off.

By talking to someone, I could strip things back. I talked about the illness. I talked about my daughter Faith's own illness. I went back to my childhood, why I had been so disruptive and the relationship with my dad that that disruption had caused. My counsellor could see I had held things in for too long, dealing with them internally when so much of it needed to be out.

I'm not saying that I am suddenly an open book, wanting to talk about every emotion that comes my way, but my experiences in recent years have helped me see a bigger picture, and I no longer have a natural impulse to store everything so deeply. My son, Devante, in his twenties and a pro footballer, is like me. I am so proud of him, but I can now look him in the eye and say, 'Don't be like your old man.'

By that I mean, don't keep things so close to your chest. Devante, like me, is a man of few words. He's very much his own man, but I can now advise my son and tell him not to let things fester. It's dangerous and unhealthy, and I learnt the hard way. Store and blow. That's what I used to do. Not any more.

So now I am starting from scratch. It's like I'm fourteen again. Back then I packed a kitbag and left my Nottingham home and, as a new Arsenal player, I headed for the FA's National School and took my eager first steps into what I hoped was the start of a brilliant football career. My drive and single-mindedness gave me so much in the game, but today, unlike my fourteen-year-old self, I don't look too far ahead and my ambitions are far simpler. Take my medication, enjoy my beautiful children, work hard, get through the day.

What will happen next? Who knows, but what I do know is that, so far, it's been a hell of a ride . . .

2

RESPECT TO MY ELDERS

I've always challenged authority. As you read my book you'll notice just that, and as I look back on my life I can see that, from as far back as I can remember, if I feel I'm being wronged, I stand up for myself. It's got me in trouble. There are plenty of relatives, teachers, team-mates, coaches and managers who would vouch for that. Their demands, their requests, their efforts to try to mould me – there were times they didn't sit well with me, and on those occasions I made my feelings clear.

This is by no means an apology. There's no point in me saying sorry to everyone. I can't change who I was. It's how I was wired. It's what made me the footballer I was. Week after week, I'd face central defenders hell-bent on making pretty studlike patterns across my shins and ankles, and to me those defenders were figures of authority. They'd push, they'd shove, they'd kick, they'd do anything they could – inside and outside the law – to make sure that they came out on top, and I treated them with the disdain I thought they deserved. I saw them as people to rage against, and that brought me success.

Now, in my late forties, I have had to treat my illness with a similar approach. To me, the illness is an authority figure: a manager trying to bully me; a coach trying to run me until I drop; a centre-back, studs up, ready to batter me. I have to take on my illness, question it, get goalside of it, convince it that when it comes to my future, *I'm* making the decisions.

On and off the pitch, I got a buzz off wanting to do things my way. It was the fuel that got my juices flowing. I can safely say that without the rebellious streak I was born with, I would never have made it to football's peaks, and so because of that, I wouldn't change a thing.

No, this is no apology, but I can look back on my life and recognise the angry young man I was and how my actions from a young age shaped me as a footballer. I can acknowledge how difficult I must have made it for so many people in my life. I also now see – with no little irony – that, despite my distrust of authority figures, my life was consistently helped by my elders and by genuine people who saw I had a talent for football and did everything they could to make sure that it didn't go to waste.

If I am going to start talking about my childhood and authority, I have to start with my dad. My old man was the master of my house and the most dominant figure in my young life. Mine was a typical Caribbean household, a culture and a place where the words 'Wait till your father gets home' were met with the fear they deserved.

Where I grew up and in the culture I came from, dads were the disciplinarians. They worked hard (and my old man worked so hard) and with that they demanded certain things. Respect was one, good behaviour was another. In the main, Dad got both, but when it came to me, the latter was hard to come by.

I was born naughty. I can't explain why I was like that, but of all of my parents' kids, I was by far the most difficult, and it affected my relationship with my dad. There's no doubt about that. He was a man of very few words and I was a boy who was unable to be still; it was a recipe for trouble and it meant that for years he and I struggled to be close.

My old man was a miner. That might surprise some people. There is not much written about the thousands of immigrants who came to England and worked underground in the pits, but that's what Dad did. I'd never really thought about it as a young man, but there is such a connection between the coal-mining industry and football.

In Scotland, legends such as Sir Matt Busby, Bill Shankly and Jock Stein all came from mining stock, and even spent their formative years working the rich seams below the ground on which they grew up. In England, Bob

Paisley was from a mining community, Bobby Robson too; Brian Clough was the son of a miner, as was the man who gave me my big break in football, Kevin Keegan.

When I was young, such thoughts didn't cross my mind. I was living in Nottingham, in my own little bubble, eating the food my dad worked hard to put on the table, without really thinking about what he was doing.

Even if I had been curious, my dad kept everything close to his chest. His young son asking him questions about his day would have been met with silence. Kids in Caribbean homes back then spoke when they were spoken to, and that was that.

I'm claustrophobic, I hate tight spaces, but that was the environment Dad worked in every day. Was he claustrophobic? I have no idea. All I know is, he went to work, toiled for hours in what must have been hard conditions and came home for some peace and quiet. With me for a son, he didn't always get it.

Both my parents came from Jamaica. Dad had met Mum there, and when she moved to England in the late 1950s with her father, my dad soon joined them. Like so many, he was sold a dream. This was the *Windrush* generation, tempted from their paradise homes with the promise of a new world, where the streets were paved with jobs, a few quid and acceptance.

Dad arrived in London, but it was Nottingham that he was headed for, to be with my mum and her father.

Work-wise, London might have offered more opportunity, but having fallen for my mum in the Caribbean, Dad was always going to follow them and it wasn't long before he was working in one of the then many coal mines in the area.

You could argue that working in the pits was better for my dad and the Caribbean men working alongside him because underground everyone is black. Dad quite recently helped with an article for the *Guardian* in which he talked about his life as a miner, underlining the fact that post-war Britain was built by so many different nationalities, from eastern Europe to the West Indies, and that in fact the Gedling Colliery in Nottinghamshire was famous for its diverse workforce.

'I enjoyed mining, because you got to make friends,' he said in the article. 'If a finger got crushed, there would be somebody there to come and give you a helping hand.' It was a unity and togetherness that my old man's generation found harder to find in the cold light of day above ground, but as a boy growing up, I only knew togetherness.

I grew up in Lenton, in south Nottingham, and my parents, myself and seven siblings eventually moved into a terraced house. It was tight, very tight, but the house was full of activity, the smells of my mum's beautiful cooking and the sound of old reggae music. Sunday was all about church and Sunday school, but as everyone on the street was so close, doors would be left open and we kids would move from home to home. My parents' best friends lived next door and the kids were all close, so there was a real sense of community.

My street had Caribbean families, white families, Asian. It was very multicultural and I never experienced any form of racism growing up. In fact, it would take football to introduce me to that nasty side of life, but for me as a boy in Lenton, a person's colour wasn't an issue at all.

My old man might have a different outlook on things. As I say, he's a man of few words, but I do recall a story he once told me about the day he arrived in London from Jamaica. He got off the boat with a short-sleeved shirt on his back and a bag of belongings. It was Baltic cold, and he headed to an address in the city he'd been given and the name of a contact who might have some work for him.

He got to the address, knocked on the door. A white woman opened the door and told Dad that his contact was not here. Dad was a bit confused and disorientated and this woman said he could leave his bag at those lodgings but he wasn't welcome. His bag was welcome but not him. That's hard to comprehend. *No Irish, No Blacks, No Dogs.* Dad would tell that story very calmly, and as I got older I couldn't understand how.

He had thought he was coming to a country that would welcome him with open arms. This was a generation that left their lives behind. They left paradise for the promise of work and a better life, but instead he found intolerance and prejudice. Jamaica wasn't only paradise because of the blue skies and turquoise seas. Dad had grown up in a place where the colour of someone's skin didn't matter, but here he was being told that a certain building wasn't accessible to him, because of just that. How can anyone be prepared for that?

I know that in those early years in England, black men would be encouraged to stay in after dark, in fear of Teddy boy gangs with chains looking for trouble. Some fought back, of course, and there were even riots – including in Nottingham – but on the whole it must have been a strange experience for so many who now called England home.

Those years here might have gone some way to forming Dad's opinion of football. He had no time for the game. Didn't understand it. Didn't want to. By the time I was growing up in the late 1970s, there were a handful of black footballers, but it wasn't easy for them, and to my dad this was not a world in which a black man should make his living. I remember saying once that I wanted to play professionally and it was met with a flat 'No'.

To him, it was the white man's game. It was the white

man's world. From the teams to the terraces, football was no place for us. 'No black man plays football,' he'd say. I tried to explain that there were black players playing for England, but he was having none of it. This was a place black men weren't allowed, a place they shouldn't want to go and an environment his son should have no ambitions about entering.

Cricket? Now that was different. Dad had, of course, been brought up watching cricket in Jamaica. He had grown up watching black men excel at it. He had watched with more than a little satisfaction as Garfield Sobers knocked English bowlers out of English grounds, and by the time I was growing up, the likes of Clive Lloyd, Viv Richards and Michael Holding would tour England in front of massive crowds who brought a touch of calypso to England's provinces. Yes, if his son was going to be a sportsman, it would be cricket.

I can remember the summers as a boy. They were long and they were hot. The smell of Caribbean cooking, that reggae music playing, Mum's food and the very real knowledge that if the West Indies were on the telly, and Richie Benaud's voice had come on the TV – 'Morning, everyone. Beautiful morning here at Trent Bridge' – you had to shut up. Oh my God, if you made a noise when the cricket was on, you took a bad whooping.

Whoopings, beatings, whatever you want to call them – like reggae and cricket, they were simply a part of my childhood. I'm not making light of the fact, beating kids is a serious issue, but the truth is, for me and so many first-generation Caribbean children, taking a beating when you did something wrong was just part of being a kid. A belt, a shoe, a slap, it's just how it was. That might sound harsh to younger people, but your dad was also your disciplinarian and you had better get used to it.

You got your ordinary love from your mum and siblings. My mum might step in if it got too bad, and on more than one occasion, knowing how angry my dad would be with me after some new misdemeanour, she would come to me and simply say, 'Hide.'

But dads showing love and affection? Are you mad? It was up to the father in the home to mould his kids. No outsider had a say, no one could step in and say, hold on, that's too much. No, if I had done something wrong, and I did quite a lot wrong, it was left for my dad to deal with me. You took it and hopefully you learnt your lesson. Or not, in my case!

Now I am a dad myself, I realise and appreciate my father, and the love he gave us all. It didn't come in the form of hugs or kisses. His words might have been few, but they were considered and everything he said to us was only ever helpful. Dad worked hard; he worked to feed us and he taught us by example. All my dad's kids have a great work ethic and we all love and respect him so much.

Looking back, though, I was a naughty kid. To be fair, in a Caribbean home, it doesn't take much to be labelled naughty. A boy fidgeting or talking to his elders when not spoken to might be seen as trouble, but for me there was no getting away from it, I was naughty. My parents must have wondered what was wrong with me and so a good smack was often the last resort.

I'm not being a victim here. It was what it was, a cultural and generational norm, and I want to reiterate that the house I grew up in was full of love. I had five older sisters and one younger one, and they, along with my mum, doted on me. Everything was done for me. The love I got from my sisters was crazy.

My mum, too, she is a wonderful woman. She accepted my dad's actions as she no doubt had grown up in a similar way. There was her cooking, so delicious, so Caribbean, and her very loving nature, but I have learnt she also was very strong-willed, a trait that I certainly inherited and one that probably explains my reluctance to let people disrespect me.

My aunts have since told me that when she was growing up, my mum would always fight her corner, never backing down, doing as she saw fit. As my mother, she didn't have to show that side of her character, but it was there and, as I say, it goes a long way to explaining my own strength of will, a will that got me into big trouble, growing up.

I got up to all sorts as a kid, answering back, disruptive stuff in a classroom, normal boyish stuff. But then there were times when I crossed the line. When I set the science lab on fire, for instance. Don't ask me why, but one day, bored, I cut the tube on the Bunsen burner, turned on the tap, sparked it up and, kaboom!, a plume of fire shot out and everything went up in flames. It was a stupid act. Other kids were in the room. My God, the teacher went mad. I was suspended, of course, and sent home, knowing that the words 'Wait till your father gets home' were soon going to be burning my ears.

My dad was of the opinion that we kids went to school and if the teacher said jump, we asked how high. School was just an extension of home. Like your parents, the teacher was always right and, having brought fire to the school, I came home knowing I was in big trouble. What a beating I took that night. Oh, I took some licks.

My dad must have wondered what to do with this tearaway son of his. By then it was only sport that was keeping me from being deemed a lost cause. Dad had made sure his love of cricket was passed down to me and I was good at it. Very good. A natural, even. I took to it so easily. Batting and bowling. That made my dad very happy and he could envisage seeing his son make a career of it. I played for Nottinghamshire schools, sailing through county trials, but then one day I had had enough. 'I don't want to play cricket,' I said, and that was that.

It just wasn't for me. I knew deep down that football was the sport I would excel at, and playing cricket, my old man's sport, was just going to get in the way. That threw him. He could see that I was stubborn; he could see that I wasn't going to back down, that this ambition of mine was very real. To him, though, there were too many obstacles in my way and he no doubt wanted to protect me from what he believed would lead ultimately to disappointment.

'You're going to have to be twice the player,' he'd say. 'No, make that three times the player than the white kid next to you.'

Looking back, they were wise words and went a long way to explaining just how strong-willed I was as I stepped into the hard world of professional football. He was right, I would have to be better and I wasn't going to let people tell me I wasn't.

In my family, the person who took the most joy from my first steps into the game was my grandad, Vincent. Vincent was a massive part of my life, a father figure, who was always giving me advice, telling me to knuckle down, urging me to keep out of trouble. I might not have listened to everything he said but I loved having his input in my life.

He was always there. Grandad would call family

meetings if there was something not right. He saw himself as the cornerstone of the clan. Now, my dad might not have seen eye to eye with him, and would often not show up to these meetings, but I always felt that Vincent wanted to be the perfect grandad, and I wish he was still around to tell him he was.

He would come and watch matches. He never pretended to understand the game but you could see the buzz he got from seeing his grandson play well and score goals. Vincent loved Brian Clough, he loved the bravado of this outspoken young manager, beating the big names around Europe. I think he reminded him of Muhammad Ali! 'You have to play for Nottingham Forest,' he used to say to me.

My mum always said that, from before I can remember, I had a ball at my feet. At night that ball was in my arms as I slept. Kids would have footballs as toys but mine seemed to be part of me. I wouldn't let go of it, always kicking it against a wall, playing with it, even in the house.

Dad, as I have explained, had no time for football and didn't want to try and understand the sport, but as I got older, got better at it, started to progress and play for a few clubs, he liked it more and more. Not because he was falling for it, but because during the weekends he knew exactly where I was, and that if I was playing football, I couldn't be getting up to anything even more unsavoury. I couldn't be on the street.

Much of our time as kids was spent outside. The park was a five-minute walk from ours and we would stay there for hours. We'd play football on the street, using a lamp post as a goalpost and a kerb as a team-mate, but it was on the park, playing games from morning to night, that we'd spend most of those long summers.

You got to know all the kids in your area, and as a young boy, aged about twelve, I would play against the bigger lads, the sixteen year olds, in games that not only helped me with my football but also introduced me to a bunch of young men who would play a big part in my life.

I was good at football, and these lads could see that. At that age, we were having too much fun to know it, but our options later in life were limited. My elders in the area in which I grew up could see my talent and they looked out for me. They were fearless and they had my back every day.

These were young guys themselves – many would go off the rails, ending up in and out of jail – but whatever nonsense they were getting up to, they made sure that I wasn't involved. That didn't please me at the time, of course, as I wanted to be seen as one of them, but no, they weren't having it. They knew I had a temper, they knew I could easily be led astray, but instead they made a decision that this kid was going to be OK.

'Andy,' they'd say, 'you've got something. We aren't allowing that to be wasted.'

I'll never forget them for that. Today, there is a lot written about gang cultures in this country. It is true that there is a very dark side to that culture, and the modern problem of knives is very real and worrying. What I grew up with wasn't like that, but it was very close to what would be thought of as a gang.

There was a sense of belonging, a sense that you stood up for each other and for the area in which you lived. We all have paths and I would never judge any of them for the path on which their lives travelled. I know that if it hadn't been for many of them, I could well have gone down the same, troubled route. It was almost inevitable. Instead, with their guidance, I was able to let my talent rather than my circumstances dictate my future.

If I viewed those guys as almost family, my actual family were also looking out for me. My sisters in particular. As was my sister's husband, another elder who saw too much in me to let it go to waste. I will always be grateful to them and to him.

I once had an altercation with a teacher at my secondary school. That was a common enough occurrence, but this one got out of hand and I was suspended for it. I was about thirteen at the time, and I went home wondering if I could style it out. Could I get away with this? I'd been excluded for single days and had managed to get away with that. Perhaps I could pretend to go to school, even creeping back into the house, unless Dad was working nights and was in sleeping all day.

This time, though, the teacher sent my parents a letter. A letter! I walked in and my dad had read it and I knew. I knew I was in trouble and I was right. He hit the roof. I took a hell of a beating and something went inside me. The lights went out. I was so angry, more angry than I had ever been, and it was all directed at that teacher.

Enraged, I left the house and I headed towards the school. I swear if I had seen him, I would have absolutely battered him. I remember thinking, 'What I just took from my dad, you're gonna get some too.' I was lucky, though. We both were. My sister had realised what was going on. She understood where I was going and followed me, catching up with me just as I walked through the school gates. 'No, you can't do this,' she said. It took her and a load of her mates to get me out of there, and I'll never forget about it because I was about to do real harm, to my teacher and to my future.

I was very lucky and I can see that. I had great support. Older boys looking out for me, older sisters understanding my emotions and knowing how to talk me down from them. There was this voice inside my head, a voice that for some reason was trying to urge me to go the other way, to take that troubled path, but I had these people nudging me, keeping me on the right track.

The incident with the teacher and that beating I took from my dad proved to me that my dad and I couldn't continue to live together for much longer. 'Two bulls in one pen' was the Caribbean term my mum used to describe us. I was only a teenager and, of course, I couldn't move out, but by now my ability with a football had given me a very real option.

It had been at primary school that my apparent ability to play football was first noticed. Mr Wilson was my teacher. Most footballers have a Mr Wilson figure in their story and he, on our concrete playground with the ball zipping across the surface, spotted that I had talent. I was always scoring goals. There weren't many other very good players, so maybe I was an easy jewel to notice, but he took a big interest in me and encouraged me to play with older boys.

On to secondary school and I was far from fazed by being at the bigger school. I was used to being around older kids, but I do remember thinking to myself, 'Keep your nose clean, stay out of trouble.' That, of course, would be easier said than done.

It was that problem with authority that would follow me into football. I didn't like these teachers and the power I perceived they had over me. Being told off by a teacher would stop me in my tracks. Being told what to do would rile me and I'd lash out. 'Are you really talking to me like that?' I'd say, and an argument would follow.

I must have been a nightmare to teach but again, and for reasons I struggle to understand, there were great teachers who persevered with me. Mr Knox and Mr Springer were my sports teachers; they looked out for me, maybe driven by the fact that the school had very few good footballers. And Mr Duckett was my head of year, a teacher who had plenty of opportunities to wash his hands of me. How I wasn't expelled, I don't know. Maybe I was a lovable rogue?

Thanks to these teachers and others around me, I could get my head down and really concentrate on my football. As well as my school, I played for my brother's team. My brother is ten years older than me, so, aged only thirteen, I was playing with and against men. Opponents didn't believe I was so young, not because of my size – I was always slight – but because I could handle their challenges. Of course, if I was ever on the end of anything too physical, and I often was, my big brother and his mates were always on hand to take care of the culprit. As I say, always someone looking out for me.

I also played for a local team called Padstow United, again with older kids and with another coach who went out of his way to look after me, driving me to and from matches and constantly encouraging me. There was also a team called JCS Garages, a local feeder team for Nottingham Forest. Two games on a Saturday, district in the morning, Padstow in the afternoon and a game on Sunday for JCS. I loved it and I couldn't stop scoring.

It wasn't long before professional clubs were taking a look. Aston Villa, Sheffield Wednesday, Chelsea – they all came to watch me, but I was too young to sign anything. For a while it looked as though my local club, Nottingham Forest, would be where I ended up.

I met Brian Clough while playing there. As a boy, I actually supported Manchester United but was well aware at a young age that, under the genius of Clough, my hometown was one of Europe's footballing hotspots. That level of success had dropped once I started having some involvement there in the early 1980s, but Clough was still this incredible presence and a manager I wish I'd played for, but as a kid, there was an incident that made me think this wasn't the place for me.

Aged around thirteen, I was in the corridor at the Forest training ground and a senior pro shouted, 'Oi, Chalky.' I have mentioned that racism hadn't been on my radar growing up. Now, at a famous football club,

I was subject to that! I didn't answer him, but of course I knew that 'Chalky' was a derogatory term, and definitely not the name my mum had given me. 'Oi, Chalky!' came the shout again. No, I'm not even going to respond. Inside I was fuming.

That was life in football, though, back then. Senior pros could say what they liked and, as a young black player, if you wanted to get on and make progress, you had better get your head down and brush it off as banter. Kick up a fuss and then the talk starts: 'Oh, he's got an attitude,' and 'Oh, he's a troublemaker.' It wouldn't be long before that sort of talk would cloud my young career, but for now I made the quick decision that Forest wasn't the club for me.

I was confident. Confident enough to leave a big First Division club who only a few years earlier were the best in Europe. If figures like Brian Clough make it clear that they think you have what it takes to make it, then, yes, you start to back yourself.

I had also been selected to join the Football Association's National School at Lilleshall. I was seen as being among the best sixteen in the country in my age group. It was another boost to my ego, and it meant that at the age of fourteen I would be leaving home to finish my studies and receive what the FA considered the best coaching a young footballer could hope for.

I backed myself to go all the way, but I was far from arrogant. I might have been stepping out into the world alone, but I was at the beck and call of the inner voices in my head. The devil and the angel, constantly at odds with each other.

Leaving for Lilleshall, I in no way thought my football career was a cert. I knew myself too well for that. I knew that I could go off the rails at any time. The possibility of me self-destructing was a very real one. The fact that I would proceed to walk out on two clubs early in my career tells you I had every right to worry.

For now, it was time to go. It was time to leave my dad. One of the bulls was leaving the pen. For all his mistrust and misunderstanding of football, Dad was pleased to see me making something of myself. Ours had been a very hard relationship, one that neither of us could mend easily, but one that softened over the years.

My dad was a man of his time. His own parents were distant with him and so it was never going to be easy for us, especially as I was never far from trouble. I regret that we were not closer back then, but today we are good. He's my old man and I love him.

In footballing terms, Dad has been an ever-present in my life, a constant, and even at the age of forty-seven, when I talk to him, there is due reverence. Aged fourteen, I was cocky, nervous and excited. I was leaving my home, but if I thought the tough love I had received from my old man was hard to handle, then the murky world of football had plenty of shocks in store for me.

3

THEY'RE GUNNING FOR ME

The Arsenal Stadium. The most special of old places.
It takes your breath away. I'm a teenager, a footballer.
I play for the Arsenal. Well, I don't play as much as I'd
like, but I have that famous crest on a blazer at home
and I'm desperate to get into the first team. The best
team in England.

The Arsenal Stadium. I'm standing outside that
famous main entrance. The uniformed doorman, the
big, black imposing doors, the art deco AFC crest, the
cannon. I walk in. The marble halls, the bust of Herbert
Chapman, the grandfather of the football club. I've been
summoned to see the current manager, George Graham.
He hardly ever talks to me, but now I've upset one of
his staff and he wants to see me, in his office. Bloody
hell.

I look at that bust. Herbert Chapman, the son of a
miner. I'm the son of a miner. Will that help me out?
No one here even knows that about me. Oh well, time
to face the music. I scale the big staircase and walk
along the wood-panelled corridor. Portraits of past

chairmen and esteemed board members hang on those walls, gazing at me disapprovingly as I make my way to the manager's office. I knock on the door and walk in. There's George. He isn't happy.

I may be a confident young footballer, but I'm awestruck by these surroundings. I won't show it, though. I sit down and immediately realise that George is slightly elevated. His desk is raised so that I'm looking up at him. Is this some sort of leadership technique? I'm a bit confused, but then he starts talking and things get even worse.

He tells me I've upset Pat Rice again and goes into this rant. 'Ya think ya the beesnees, din't ya?'

George has a broad Glaswegian accent and I don't understand what he is on about.

'Excuse me?' I ask.

'You, ya think ya the beesnees, din't ya?'

I'm nodding away, not knowing what the hell 'beesnees' is, making him angrier and angrier.

'Ya fancy yoursel' as a big-time player, din't ya?'

'I think I'm half decent, yeah.'

'You think you're the bloody beesnees.'

Oh, he means the bee's knees!

'Get out!' he says.

Not a problem for me. He's the one who asked me in there. I walk back down those grand corridors, down the imposing staircase, past Mr Chapman, and I'm filling with rage. I don't care where I am, or who he is, why's he talking to me like that? I step out through those doors and down the steps and onto the street. Standing there, I know. I know that I'll never play for George Graham's Arsenal again.

Arsenal Football Club came to my home in Nottingham on my fourteenth birthday. Terry Murphy was there at the door, the club's chief scout. Like the club itself, he was always immaculately turned out. Club blazer and tie, an old-school football man who said all the right things to both me and my parents. Where do I sign?

Schoolboy forms taken care of, I travelled to the National School at Lilleshall an Arsenal scholar and nervously excited about where I was heading. Not that excitement was always the overriding emotion. Having got through the first trial, I had given a false address to the guy who was picking me up for the second. I didn't want to go. I wasn't that bothered. The thing is, this guy called my home wondering where I was and my mum was angry, as she hated lateness. It was bad manners to have left this guy waiting, and while I made some excuse, they arranged for me to be collected and I was off for the next trial. I once again impressed and I was selected.

Lilleshall is a daunting place. A big, old, grand

building in Shropshire. Think Hogwarts for young, sporting wizards. It was like nothing I'd ever seen before. As I said goodbye to my mum and my brother, who had driven, I, like the other boys, was suddenly alone. It was hard, but you had to cope. We trained, we went to the local school to study, but there was so much more to handle.

We were kids away from home for the first time, but this was not an institution interested in warmth. There was a nice old couple that looked after us, but I had never been away from my family for more than two days, and now two years stretched ahead of me. Being kids, we didn't say much. You could see that lots of them were struggling, but you just got on with things, trying not to show a weakness.

It was going to get very tough, though. Overwhelming, even. For a long time, I would wake up disoriented, wondering where I was, wondering why I wasn't at home. Sixteen boys deemed the best footballers in their age group. Sixteen boys in the year above us. Ian Walker was there, who would play for Tottenham and England. Bryan Small, who played for Aston Villa, became a big pal. We had the blazer and tie emblazoned with the Three Lions. I wasn't that fussed about all that, it didn't mean much to me then, and anyway it quickly became clear that there were far bigger things to think about.

From the off, the boys were jostling for position.

You'd be looking around, studying the other boys playing in your position. And then there were the older boys. Within the first ten days or so, they let me know that there would be an initiation. They wouldn't tell you when it would happen but it was coming. Let's see what these young boys are all about.

Our group's 'initiation' came in the dead of night. We were in our beds, in our dormitory, when the door was flung open and in came a group of older lads. By the time we had sat up, startled and terrified, they were on us. Bang. You'd better get up on your feet and fight back. Lie down and take the beating and you're seen as the boy with no heart. You had to give it back. I did. I was used to fighting, but this was nasty.

Bars of soap and shoes wrapped in pillowcases. It was like a scene from a borstal movie. There was blood and there were tears. Done with us, the older boys left us to cry into our pillows and that was that. Let's see who fancies this – that was the thought process, but it was simply bullying. Let's see who's got balls and let's see who's a bit milky. I don't know if the adults there knew about it, but I would guess they did. It was a tradition. As second-years we did it to the new lads, and on and on it went.

I had fought back against those attackers, and the irony was I then began to be supported by them. They saw that I could give it, that I was a fighter and that I might go far. Within six months, I got on with most of the older boys, and once I became a second-year, you simply learnt to test the new crop in the same way.

The actual football side of things was OK. Dave Sexton was in charge of the coaching and he was good. Very matter-of-fact, though, and I would say, looking back, that the methods were a bit too professional. We were kids, remember. Fourteen and fifteen, but there was no fun element. All very methodical and precise. Yes, we learnt lots, but where was the individuality? Where were the surprises, the off-the-cuff stuff? I just think it could have been more fun.

The academic school we all attended was far from fun, too. It was a mixed local comprehensive and us footballers had to stick together because there was always trouble waiting around the corner. 'Why are you talking to our birds?' we'd be asked. There would be racial slurs too and you made sure you didn't walk around alone too much. If anything, it made us players closer.

Over the two years, there were loads of occasions when I'd had enough. Loads of times, especially in the first two or three months, my bag was packed. I missed my home, my family, but I also missed the close-knit community in which I had grown up. I had loads of conversations with my brother, who would talk me down, saying, 'Why come home, mate? You have to work at it. You have to stick at it. What have you got to come back to?'

At my lowest, I could answer that last question with the simple answer 'I have my family to come back to.' I knew that wasn't right, though. I wanted to succeed *for* my family. Everything I ever achieved was for them, and so deep down I knew my brother was right and I would unpack and crack on.

I didn't tell my sisters or my parents how hard it was at Lilleshall. I kept that in. Maybe I was becoming more and more like my dad, but when I left the National School at sixteen, I had changed. I was different. I had had to grow up, that's for sure. The naughty kid who had left had gone. I understood I had responsibilities, that I was now a man, but there was more to it than that.

I was harder. More distant from my family. I had always been very lovable with my sisters. Laughing with them, draping myself over them on the living-room sofa, accepting their affection, but now I wore a mask at home. I had discovered how hard the world of football was and how hard the path ahead of me was going to get. I didn't want to worry them about it, I didn't want them to share my concerns.

*

Don't get me wrong, I was more than up for it and moved down to Arsenal hungrier than ever to succeed. My mum was happy because one of my sisters now lived in London and I could stay with her. I wasn't fazed by being in the capital. I felt at home. We lived in Edmonton and then Enfield in north London, and so it was ideal for training.

I was desperate to play. Arsenal had sold themselves to me on their record for promoting youth-team players. The proof was everywhere you looked. The first team was full of young talent, most of it scouted by Terry Murphy and developed by a club willing to give youth its chance. Michael Thomas, Paul Merson, David 'Rocky' Rocastle, Paul Davis. Tony Adams was made captain. Niall Quinn, Martin Hayes, they were all playing. David O'Leary was the older pro, but he'd come through the ranks. It was the perfect environment for a young footballer to know he could thrive, the perfect education.

During half-terms and holidays from the National School, I used to come to Arsenal's London Colney ground to train and if I was eating my lunch, the first-team squad would always fire into me. Come and chat. It was clear they had taken an interest in me. Maybe they'd heard good things about me; maybe they felt they were like me, I don't know. I must admit to being cautious. My natural scepticism had me wondering what these guys wanted, what was in it for them, but I think the likes of Rocky and Mickey Thomas were from similar backgrounds as me and they understood me.

I took it all in. I watched these guys closely in pre-season games and in friendlies. I was aspiring to be where they were. I was aspiring to be just like them. In fact, I felt I already was. I had to keep myself in check. *Don't blow this*. I had got through the hardship of Lilleshall without blowing it, but I couldn't relax. That self-destruct button was still there, waiting to be pressed at any time.

For a start, I had to check my thoughts about the boss. George Graham strutted about the place and I didn't know what to make of him. He was having himself, though. Properly having himself. If he was chocolate he'd have taken a bite. I remember looking at him. I was a kid, he was the manager, and yes I was in awe. I wanted to impress him, I wanted to know he'd noticed me, but one day he might say, 'Good mornin', son,' and some days, most days, nothing. He was one of those.

My opinion of the main man was set early, and it wouldn't be long before he had made up his mind about me. Stay out of trouble? Me? No chance. My first fall-out with the club was over my pro contract. I was a Youth Trainee. Pro contracts were given out at eighteen but I discovered that some of the Scottish and Irish boys were signing theirs at seventeen. That was not right. I was fuming. They were mugging me off.

I couldn't stay silent about it. Impossible. I went to see the youth-team manager, Pat Rice, and Terry Murphy. I told them how I felt, I let them know. I went into one. How come these guys are getting pro contracts? Why not me? I was impatient. They tried to explain that they needed to ensure that the players from outside of England signed, but I wasn't having it.

There it was. I felt that these people, people of authority, were dictating my life. I felt that they and their rules were being imposed on me and I let them know. News would filter up to George. Talk was spreading: 'Andy Cole has an attitude problem.'

From then on, it felt like someone was always questioning me and my young methods, that the eyes of the club's hierarchy were on me, perhaps waiting for me to mess up and confirm their suspicions. Ricey was doing his best for me, but I did feel that the club were trying to change me. Football back then had this preconception about us black players (in fact it still does). It might have been a subconscious thing, but it was there. If a young white player kicked up a fuss, he had spirit. If a young black player did the same, he was labelled a troublemaker. I truly believe that.

I also understand how frustrating it must have been for Pat and some of his staff. They saw a good footballer, but – with their old-school beliefs – they felt the best way to cure my apparent problems was to get on my case. And so, when I trained with the youth team, they were on me. Every day.

I was a terrible trainer. Throughout my career I struggled to put in the 110 per cent required by the English game. This, they felt, had to be rubbed out of me. One day, Ricey was particularly frustrated. '******* hell, Coley, you're like a ******* lighthouse.'

Tired of his constant shouting, I cracked. I had had enough. I walked off. I can't have people talking to me like that. I walked off, straight into the dressing room, showered and left. I remember Paddy O'Leary was giving me a lift to the tube station that day and he was great, trying to understand me, not judging but offering advice.

I wasn't in the mood to listen, though. I got to my sister's, packed my bag, explained to her what had happened and headed back to Nottingham. 'It's not for me,' I said to her as I left. I meant it too. I was finished with football. It had proved too much even for someone like me, apparently able to cope with a harsh environment. Maybe those experiences at Lilleshall that I had kept bottled up had fizzed to the surface, but for a couple of days I was done. 'People can't talk to me like that or treat me like that,' I said to my family.

*

As the dust settled, Arsenal were in touch again. Calling my home, talking to my family. Saying the right things. They promised me that pro contract on my eighteenth birthday. I already missed the football and so I returned to London, telling myself again to keep my head down, to stay out of trouble. Now, though, my employers also knew all about my self-destructive streak.

I was lucky. I had been given a second chance at a club where so many senior pros seemed to have taken to me. They showed genuine interest in me, especially those who had come through the ranks. Paul Davis was great. Pops, as we called him, would take me to one side, knowing what had happened, and really try to get through to me.

'Andy, what are you doing?'

'Nothing, Pops. I'm just getting on with things.'

He wouldn't let it lie, though, and would stay on my back.

'Do you know how much talent you have?' he'd ask. 'You have to sort your head out. Causing problems around here, with the gaffer, that's going to stop you getting where you need to be.'

I listened and I appreciated what he was saying, but at my worst I didn't care. I was a young man raging. A young man fighting some sort of invisible battle. The more I was pushed into doing something, the more I would dig in and fight that way of thinking.

Rocky and Mickey were the same. They would take me with them on nights out. I was still a youth-team player, scoring goals for the reserves, yes, but still, these were Arsenal players, England players, the best around, and they were looking out for me. I had to fight the urge to distrust them, to wonder what was in it for them, but I'll never forget their generosity and the belief they showed in me.

Talking of belief, Ricey must have seen a responsible side to me, because at one point he made me foreman in the youth team. Foreman meant that I was in charge of all the duties and would allocate jobs to my young team-mates. Dressing rooms, floors, cleaning boots, sorting the kits – it all had to be done and I was in charge. Yes, I hated it.

Remember that I was used to my sisters clearing up after me and my dislike of cleaning back then was matched by my dislike of telling people what to do. I was far from the diligent boss. A team-mate would tell me he'd finished, and I'd just say, nice one, see you later. Ricey would then walk in, run his finger along the still-dirty surface, and make me do it again. Are you taking the mickey?

Young footballers, of course, don't have to do all that any more, and people think the game is lesser for it. I'm not sure. I hated it. People say it's character-building. How is it character-building? With me, it just caused more friction. I'd play with the reserves on a Saturday, do well, score goals, and then afterwards the dressing-room floor that me and my team-mates had *all* walked on was dirty and I was the one who had to clean it. What's that about?

I can look back now and laugh at how much I hated all that, but the truth is, little by little, and with each tut and grumble, a case was being built against me, and George, for all my talent, interpreted what he saw as a problem with my attitude. If a young player was wanted for training with the senior lot, my fellow striker in the youth team, Kwame Ampadu, was almost always chosen over me.

I loved Kwame, he was a great lad. A black guy with a southern Irish accent! He always made me laugh, but we were chalk and cheese. Kwame worked his socks off. I was pleased for him when he would get his chance, but I could see it came down to attitude over ability. I was getting overlooked by George because of that chip on my shoulder, a chip that according to the staff at Arsenal was growing fatter and juicier by the day. It didn't matter to me. However much Ricey – who I do think truly believed in me – would tell me where I was going wrong, I would dig in and fight back.

The senior players who had taken to me were pulling their hair out. Looking back, I can acknowledge my faults, acknowledge that I was an angry young man, battling away against God knows what. I can't change the past, though, and therefore I have no regrets. 'You did it your way,' Paul Davis said to me later, and I guess he was right. My ambitions were on the line, though. I couldn't curb the young lad I was, and might have blown it.

What got me through was sheer ambition. Talent, too, but I was so keen to play first-team football that I thought all the problems would take care of themselves. It was a desire made even more fervent watching the first team win two league titles in three seasons. The 1989 championship-deciding game at Anfield was incredible. What scenes! My mate Mickey Thomas getting that late goal and winning it for such a young team. I thought I was in the right place.

George had built a great team. They would go on and win the title again in 1991. I always thought it was the team's organisation that saw them gain their success. I'm not being critical, George was brilliant at getting his teams as well drilled as any we'd ever seen, but considering some of the players there, I'd like to have seen a bit more flair. A bit more freedom.

Paul Merson was some footballer. A real talent, Merse could play through the middle or come off the wing and hurt teams. I liked Merse a lot. A top fella. Then there was David Rocastle. It's hard to explain to people how good Rocky was. Yes, people and fans saw him play, and saw so many great moments and goals, but there was something special about him that you only fully appreciated if you worked with him.

A south London boy, Rocky had come through the ranks and become an instant hit. He was the most popular guy at the club. Us youngsters looked up to him. I know the likes of Ian Wright, who came from the same area as him, idolised him, and his amazing generosity with his time for us young footballers was matched by the sheer skill he had with the ball at his feet.

I do believe, however, that he could have been even better. At Arsenal, Rocky was in a very structured team. Every tiny detail was worked on. The back four, the cornerstone of George's success at Highbury, was drilled to within an inch of its life. I'd look with bewilderment in training as George would have Lee Dixon, Tony, Steve Bould and Nigel Winterburn moving around together, all holding a long rope, to keep them as one unit. I mean, it worked, don't get me wrong, but that methodical approach shouldn't have applied to the likes of Rocky.

Everyone had their role and their partnerships. The right-back with the centre-half, the left-back with the left-midfield, the two central midfielders. All that is important, of course, but I would love to have seen Rocky left out of all that. Arsenal's great rivals at that time were Kenny Dalglish's Liverpool. Now, Kenny liked to organise a team too, but he also knew that in John Barnes he had a rare talent and he allowed him to roam as he pleased.

With that sort of freedom, I really believe that Rocky could have been one of the very best. I can hear George now in training: 'David!' That's all you'd hear the whole session. 'David!' In that thick Glaswegian accent. 'David, get back!' 'David, pass it!' Get back? Pass it? Rocky should have been told to get forward and beat a man with his array of tricks. Even then, I would mutter 'Leave him alone' under my breath.

I was desperate to play alongside Rocky. I'd picture him beating his full-back and crossing the ball for me to score in front of a packed North Bank, but for now I had to settle for reserve-team football in front of a maximum of a thousand loyal souls. I wasn't moaning, though. It was a great education. Proper tough.

You'd have loads of first-team players coming back from injuries and so it wasn't Mickey Mouse stuff. And the challenges? My God. You had to harden up and quickly. I learnt so much playing for the reserves. I scored loads too, and playing in front of those small crowds only got my juices flowing more. I'd score to a polite ripple of applause and quickly wanted so much more. My adrenaline was up and I couldn't wait to get out there for the first team, couldn't wait to score, couldn't wait to hear the cheers of a real crowd.

I got on as a sub against Sheffield United at Highbury over Christmas in 1990, but my chances were limited to only one more substitute appearance, this time against Tottenham at Wembley in the Charity Shield the following August. I was lively that afternoon and I'd done well in a pre-season tournament at Highbury against the likes of Sampdoria and Panathinaikos. I think there were a lot of Arsenal fans excitedly readying themselves for me joining that impressive list of talent to come through the ranks at their club.

I felt close. So close. The manager had other ideas, though. It was like having a Ferrari in your drive but no one will give you the keys. I was desperate to play, or should I say desperate to be shown there was a clear path for me, but in George I was relying on a manager who had made his mind up. To him, my attitude was such a problem that it wasn't worth being patient, it wasn't worth him putting the work in to get the very best out of me. I wasn't going to get the chance.

Even so, on the odd occasion when I was asked to join the first team for training, I used to give it my absolute all. I loved it. I would work my socks off.

Ricey must have wondered why I didn't always train like that as I tore about, getting right into Tony and Bouldy. *Show them what you're about.* The two of them would kick the hell out of me, which told me I was doing all right, and those sessions poured further petrol on the flames of my ambition. I also showed the first-team players I had a bit, and I know the likes of Merse always thought I should have got my chance at Arsenal.

I wasn't arrogant enough to think I was good enough to walk into the team. I just wanted an indication that I would get an opportunity. I thought I was already better than some of the forwards there, players like Perry Groves, but I had nothing but respect for Kevin Campbell, the striker now regularly partnering Alan Smith up front.

Not only did I respect Kevin, I looked up to him. He had come through the ranks at Arsenal, banged in the goals in the reserves and on loan at Leyton Orient and broken through, scoring plenty of goals on the way to the title in 1991. He was also a good friend.

Like so many of the players, Kevin had looked out for me at Arsenal. Taking me on nights out, making me feel very much part of the set-up. It was weird. Although I was on the periphery of things, the lads had taken to me and even in places like the first-team dressing room at Highbury, a strictly first-team habitat, I was welcomed.

Tony Donnelly, the kit man at Highbury, had a rule about the home dressing room. No youth-team players or reserves allowed unless you were doing duties. Not me. Kevin would say, Coley, you're in here with us. The night Arsenal received the 1991 league championship, I was sitting in there with the lads, having a beer, and Tony was probably thinking, 'What the hell is he doing?'

Kevin was like a big brother to me. I even met my future wife at Kevin's brother's wedding. I never ever saw Kevin as a competitor. *I* was my only big competition. Myself. That's who I was fighting against, and I certainly never saw a spot in the team as a gimme. I just wanted to play, and so, later in 1991, when the possibility of a loan deal to Fulham came up I jumped at the chance.

By this time I had had my awkward summons to George's office and got the hint that my chances in Arsenal's red and white were going to be limited. Fulham were in the old Third Division, but no matter: it was first-team football and I was desperate.

Great little club, Fulham, but at the time they were skint and, I won't lie, the transition from Arsenal's marble halls was a hard one. The training pitches were basically a park and we had to take home our training kit to wash it ourselves. This will make me sound like a spoilt, sulky young footballer, but when you're used to a meticulous kit man like Donners at Arsenal, it was a culture shock.

I struggled. The senior pros at Fulham were nowhere near as warm and helpful as those at Highbury. The likes of Ray Lewington and Chris Pike were stand-offish, tricky. My clear desire to better myself can't have helped, of course, but these guys showed no interest in making my short stay there remotely educational.

On one occasion, I could see their minds ticking, judging me. We were travelling to a game up north and the coach broke down. The players were asked to push and I refused. I wasn't pushing the bus. I know, once again I come across as the entitled young footballer, and I probably should have pushed, but the players had been so unwelcoming that I felt little for them in return. They could push their own bus. 'Who does he think he is?' I could hear them asking.

I was frustrated there. I scored a few goals but it didn't go well. Maybe I did feel it was beneath me. I had been studying the Arsenal first team so closely, and knew I was good enough to make it there, but here I was, being asked to wash kit and push buses. Yes, my young, eager self found that hard.

News about my attitude once again spread and, as with George at Highbury, I was summoned to a meeting, this time with Fulham's chairman, Jimmy Hill, in the less opulent surroundings of Craven Cottage. I hadn't met Jimmy before, but he clearly had an opinion on me, stating categorically that I wasn't the player I thought I was. 'You haven't got a chance,' were his words. I told him I thought I did and went on my way. What an ********, I thought as I walked out of the famous little building. My time at Fulham was at an end.

So was my time at Arsenal. Another loan spell beckoned, this time at Bristol City in the old Second Division. It was another opportunity to play first-team football, another chance to prove the doubters – and they were increasing in number – wrong.

Arsenal just weren't going to take the chance on me. My grandfather, a big figure in my life, always advocated going backwards to go forwards. He had left the Caribbean home he loved to come to England to better himself and provide for his family. That might have been a step back, but it eventually moved us all forward and I would take the same attitude – there's that word again – with me to the West Country in the hope that this time I would show people what I was all about.

I can look back on my time at Arsenal and acknowledge that I was difficult, but I still think the manager and his staff should have given me more of a chance.

I heard only fairly recently a rumour that Arsenal had got rid of me because I was stealing from the dressing room. God knows how these rumours start, but it's nonsense.

Nearly thirty years after I left Highbury, Arsenal fans still stop me and talk about what might have been. David Dein, the club's former chief executive, always gushes about how big a mistake it was selling me. I've seen George since, of course, and it is always amiable. 'I knew you were good enough, we just had too many good strikers,' he'll say.

In the end, George and his staff didn't think I was worth the hassle. That's fair enough. Soon, I'd be someone else's problem.

4

A ROBIN TO A MAGPIE

I love Bristol City! During my career I got my hands on the biggest and most prestigious of trophies, I played at Wembley, scored at the Nou Camp, called the likes of Eric Cantona a team-mate and Zinedine Zidane an opponent. From those days as a young kid, when I would fall asleep holding a football, I dreamt of playing on the highest stage, of scoring the goals that won the silverware. I can look back on the most dazzling of times, but it was at Bristol City, a homely club in the West Country, playing in the second tier of England's game, that I can safely say I came alive as a professional footballer.

My short time at Ashton Gate, firstly on loan, was a rocket just when my career needed ignition. It was the time that convinced people I was good enough. Before moving there, the game I presumed I loved had seemed a dark place. My loneliness in the dormitory at Lilleshall, the seemingly blocked pathway at Arsenal, the uncertainty at Fulham – it had all seemed so overcast, as if maybe it wasn't to be, but then, at Bristol City, the lights came on.

For that I have to thank Denis Smith, the manager with his finger on the switch. Denis was brilliant with me. He was old-school, very old-school, but he quickly understood how I worked. He was an old centre-half, with old beliefs, but with me, a confident young striker, he was modern and he knew how to get the best out of me. I'll always be grateful for that.

It was nice to get out of London again and even nicer to find a group of players so welcoming. I settled immediately, scoring big goals – the club were in a relegation battle at the end of the 1991–92 season – at Sunderland and Millwall, plus a few at home, in front of a crowd that quickly took to me.

It was perfect. I was playing with a smile, for a manager who liked me and rated me. Denis made it clear he wanted to sign me permanently. I thought little of that idea, reckoning there was no way Arsenal would sell. We played our last game at Watford. I scored a couple of goals and thought that was that. Time to say my goodbyes and thank-yous and be on my way.

I then got two phone calls. One was from Liam Brady, the manager at Celtic. He wanted to sign me, but Arsenal said no. OK, they want to keep me. I'll be getting my chance. Then, a couple of weeks later I had a call from Pat Rice saying Derby County had shown an interest. I was surprised he was telling me because I still thought they fancied me themselves.

'Does George want to sell me, Ricey?' I asked.

There was a long pause, and he said he'd get back to me. I never heard from Pat Rice again. I'm not sure exactly what went on. Who knows what happened to Derby's interest, but soon Arsenal were in touch, saying that they had accepted a £500,000 bid from Bristol City and I could go down to negotiate personal terms.

I didn't have an agent, so my brother came with me and on the M4 we decided I'd just listen. I wasn't going to sign anything. Listen and then leave. Understood. A couple of hours later, and with my brother's eyebrows raised, I was signing a three-year £500-a-week contract. Why wait? I liked the club, I knew the players and got on with them (most of them). I liked the manager and he liked me. Let's do it. It was one of the best decisions I ever made.

Denis said all the right things. He told me that neither he nor the club would stand in my way if a bigger club came in for me with the right offer. I wasn't thinking that far ahead, but it was nice to hear. Denis had a budget of £750,000. He'd spent two-thirds of that on me. The other £250,000 had gone on Raymond Atteveld from Everton.

The fee didn't play on my mind at all. It was a lot of money, a big amount to spend on a player yet to play much first-team football. But I was happy to be there, too happy getting up in the morning and going to work and earning a bit of money to worry about transfer fees.

It felt so positive. I had taken a knock when Arsenal had sold me, but I wasn't going to dwell on it. The writing had been on the wall at Highbury for a long time. As for the constant worries about messing things up, they had gone too. Those thoughts I'd always had – *stay out of trouble* – they'd gone. There was no need. I was content with my surroundings.

I had taken a hard route to get here, but I was moving forward. There had been so much nonsense. George, Jimmy Hill, Ricey, all with their doubts about me. A lot of it was my fault, I know that, but now I was playing for a manager who truly rated me. I was putting a bit of money into my pocket and I'd met Shirley, who was in London and was now my girlfriend. Life was sweet.

Being a footballer was never about the trappings. Never about fame or adulation. I loved the game. Loved it! If you are in it for anything other than the game, then it's all wrong. I loved taking on defenders, working, winning, coping with losing. It was all about the Saturday afternoon. Denis got that. He could see I wasn't going to be the greatest trainer. Nowhere near. But instead of trying to change me, he wanted me to be at my best on a Saturday, and if that meant saving a bit, then great. 'Just be on time, Coley,' he said to me. 'Just be on time and do your thing.' Music to my ears.

The players at City were the same. They didn't try to work me out. The staff at Arsenal wanted to change me. The pros at Fulham quickly made their minds up about me. My team-mates at City were keen to win games and they saw I was capable of helping them do just that and made me feel part of things straight away.

The attacking players were particularly accommodating. Leroy Rosenior, Wayne Allison and Dariusz 'Jacki' Dziekanowski were great with me. I had admired Leroy from afar for a long time. He'd scored goals at West Ham and was a brilliant centre-forward. Great in the air, strong, good finisher. Leroy had bad knees but was starting to think about coaching and he was always willing to pass on some good knowledge.

Wayne, or 'the Chief' as we called him, was another fine centre-forward. Strong like Leroy and just as helpful, the Chief and I worked well together. In one of my first games we were away at Sunderland and I was getting some treatment from a tough defender called John Kay. Kay didn't mess about and he kept leaving it on me.

'Don't worry about that,' Wayne said, and five minutes later, he'd splattered Kay all over the place. I'd never seen anything like it. The lad was left rolling around on the floor. The Chief just winked at me, and from there I knew I was going to be OK.

It was easy to play with these guys. If I was up front with Leroy or Wayne, it was a classic big man–little man partnership. We didn't just lump it up, though. We had good players – Mark Aizlewood, Gary Shelton, Russell Osman – all good footballers and good lads. Leroy and the Chief were good footballers, too, intelligent forwards, and I could make clever runs knowing they would find me.

Then there was Jacki Dziekanowski. Jacki was a one-off. What a player. He was loved at Celtic, and was equally as popular at Bristol City. He was one of the most skilful players I ever played with. He'd flick the ball over people's heads for fun. If Jacki could have stayed sober, he could have been anything. The big Polish forward had a real problem with drink, and not just a few too many beers: vodka. We loved him, though.

I ran into him recently and he looked so well. He'd clearly beaten his demons (we all have them) and I was so happy to see him. 'I didn't think you'd remember me,' he said as I shook his hand, but how could I have forgotten Jacki? Top, top player.

One of the guys that I didn't rate as a footballer or as a person was Ray Atteveld. My God, he rated himself. He had come from the Premier League and that's where he thought he belonged. He had the flash Mercedes and walked about like some big-time Charlie, but he was useless. 'Bobbins', as we say in football.

He was the exception, though, and training was always good, always educational and, with Denis joining in, always competitive. Denis might have been the boss, but once he was out on that training ground, he was back to being the bruising centre-half he had always been. Ouch. He'd get stuck in, hard. It added to the fun I was having there.

No one was judging me, no one was trying to get into my head or work out how to change me. I was younger than everyone and I might have had other interests, but I was accepted. With a decent wage, I was buying nice clothes and would leave the labels on the sleeves. I think a few of the older guys wondered why I'd still have a BOSS tag on a jacket or a Versace tag on a shirt. What can I say? I was a sucker for fashion.

The lads would ask me out on their nights out in Clifton – and they could drink! That wasn't really my thing, but I'd go along and have a great time. There was no bitterness towards me. Some senior pros can resent a young player making his way, being successful and looking at a career ahead of him. I had experienced that at Fulham but not at Bristol City. In this perfect environment, I could enjoy the coaching, work hard (well, as hard as I needed to) and play well. No talk of my attitude. Put it this way, if the Bristol City team bus had ever broken down, I would have been the first out there giving it a push.

I started the 1992–93 season with a hat-trick in a 5–1 League Cup win over Cardiff, with the Chief and Leroy getting a goal each. There's no love lost between City fans and Cardiff, so that was a good night for the fans, and I continued to score goals from there. Results for the team were mixed, but I was enjoying my football and my life, with little concern or thought for my future.

That season, we played in something called the Anglo-Italian Cup, a tournament for clubs outside the newly formed Premier League and our lower-league cousins in Italy. Cosenza, Pisa, Reggiana – not giants of the Italian game, but I loved the experience, pitting my skills against a very Italian way of defending. Years later, it would stand me in good stead. What I didn't enjoy was being spat at. Right in the face. I had never experienced anything like that. It was degrading, but I guess you have to take it and learn.

It was the same with the small degree of fame that my form had afforded me. People were writing nice things about me and I was recognised around Bristol. The articles in the press were never taken that seriously. I was young and, of course, it's nice to see positive headlines, but I quickly decided not to pay too much attention to the stuff I had no control over. It was an attitude that served me well later when, as a Manchester United and England player, the articles were not so kind.

The fame bit was also something I didn't much care for. The people that know me, really know me, know that I don't do limelight. I'm a quiet man by nature and comfortable around those few people I know well. I liked that my family could see I was doing well, that they could see that all the things they had done for me growing up were paying off. That's what made me happy. Anyway, Bristol was a great city, not overbearing at all, and the fans, they might stop you and offer support, but it was in no way intrusive.

The goals continued to flow and there was talk of other clubs scouting me. One day, Denis came to me and said that Nottingham Forest had put in a bid for me. My hometown club, Brian Clough. They were struggling in the Premier League's inaugural season, but, OK, that could be interesting.

Denis was nothing but open with me. He said that the offer was simply too low. I think it was about £700,000. Arsenal had put a sell-on clause in my contract (which was tight of them, I thought) and so, had City accepted Forest's bid, they would have been left with no profit at all. I totally respected Denis's stance on the matter. I wasn't going to kick off. This wasn't Denis going back on his word that he and the club wouldn't stand in my way. This was simple business and, considering what everyone had done for me, I thanked him for letting me know and got on with things.

I think Denis and his board were starting to fall out. Denis was willing to sell me if the offer was right, but some at the club were against it. With results still mixed, it came to a head and Denis was sacked. I felt for him. He had been brilliant for me and brilliant for my career, so I was naturally concerned about who would replace him.

Those concerns were immediately quashed when news broke that the club were promoting from within and appointing Russell Osman as manager. Russell was a mate and now my boss. When I arrived, he and his lovely wife, Louise, would have me over for dinner and I always appreciated their hospitality.

Oz was great. What a footballer. Part of Bobby Robson's outstanding Ipswich Town team of the early 1980s and an England centre-half. He loved to play the game right, could carry the ball out from defence, and I knew he'd make a good coach. He sat me down and reiterated that if the right offer came in, the club and any doubting board members wouldn't block a move. Soon an offer came in that even the most sceptical director simply could not refuse.

*

Newcastle United were the best team in our division. We'd gone to them in September 1992 and got beaten 5–0 and they had been flying. Most of what I knew about them was through my old mate Lee Clark, who I had played England youth football with. Clarky was a Geordie through and through and wouldn't shut up about the city, its people or the club. When there was talk of Newcastle watching me, Clarky's phone calls became more and more regular.

'Coley, get your arse up here, man,' he'd say. 'You'd love the Toon, man.'

'What's the Toon?' I'd ask naively.

I loved Slim (he was always putting on weight) and his enthusiasm was infectious, but I had my doubts. It was so far away, for a start. My girlfriend, Shirley, lived in London and so my life was Bristol, the M4 and London. I was comfortable with that sort of distance, but Newcastle? It seemed like too much.

'Forget all that, son,' Clarky would say. 'We'll take care of ya, man.'

I thought little more of it until one day when I was doing my laundry at the local laundrette (I had become very domesticated and no longer needed my mum or my sisters for that sort of thing). Having finished one load, I came out to find a note on the windscreen of my car. Not a bloody ticket, I thought, but it was from the manager: 'Coley, give me a call when you can. Oz.'

I phoned him and he told me that Newcastle had put in an offer, it had been accepted and their manager, Kevin Keegan, wanted to speak to me immediately.

'Are you sure, Oz?' I asked.

'Yes, it's a big offer.'

Kevin Keegan and Newcastle had offered £1.75 million, a figure a club like Bristol City could not turn down. Kevin called me that day but our relationship got off to an awkward start.

'Hello Adrian,' he said.

I was confused. 'Er, no, this is Andrew.' There was a pause.

'Oh, sorry, Andrew, sorry. I meant Andrew.'

It wasn't the best start, but he was very enthusiastic. 'As you know, Andrew, we've agreed a fee with Bristol City and we'd like to get you up here on the shuttle tonight.'

'I can't.'

'What, why not?' Kevin asked, probably wondering if he'd blown it by calling me Adrian.

'It's laundry day today and I have some more loads to do.'

'Er, OK. How about tomorrow?'

'Yeah, tomorrow is fine.'

It was one of the stranger conversations, but that was that. I had to get my laundry done, go to London, where I had a flat, sort myself out and get myself up to

Newcastle. It was at my flat that I received another phone call, one that would prove to me that not only was I going up in the footballing world, but that the higher you went, the more devious life got.

'Hello, Coley, it's Paul Elliott.'

I didn't know Paul personally but I knew the Luton, Pisa and Celtic footballer he'd been. My upbringing meant I always had time for my elders and so I gave him the respect he deserved.

'I hear you're going to Newcastle,' he said. 'I also hear you don't have an agent, but I can help you if you like. Steve Waggott is a great agent and he is happy to look after you.'

News had travelled fast, but fair enough. I knew no better. I'd never had an agent, but this was a big deal and maybe I would need some help. 'OK, cool. I'll meet Steve.'

We met with Newcastle and the negotiations were smoothly done. Great four-year contract, no problem. On top of that I was getting a £30,000 signing-on fee. I'd never seen money like that in my life. Now it was going in my pocket. I was buzzing.

'That signing-on fee,' Waggott said. 'That's mine.'

'You what?'

'That's my fee for doing the deal.'

Doing the deal? There had been no negotiating; it was the smoothest move ever. In my mind, all these people had done was latch on to me, convince me I needed their help and then take my money. Again, I didn't know any better, so while I was gutted to lose thirty grand, I thought, OK, he's my agent, that's how it works. The thing is, and this to me is the disgusting bit, I never heard from Waggott or Elliott again. The way I saw it, I had been robbed.

I can look back now and say I was naive. Despite good people like David O'Leary at Arsenal trying to talk me into having one, I had never had an agent of any sort before, and because Elliott was a former pro, I just took it that I'd be well looked after. Instead, I felt that I had had my pants taken down. Waggott had technically been the agent brokering my contract. There had been no negotiating as such but, OK, he was due a fee. The whole £30,000, though? I remember my new manager Kevin Keegan finding out later and being particularly surprised.

It was twenty-odd years later that I next saw Paul Elliott. I was at an event with Cyrille Regis at Wembley and Paul was in the room. Cyrille is my mentor, my hero, the pioneer for all us black footballers, and he could see that I was starting to fume. I explained what had happened, and Cyrille, the most calm and thoughtful of men, told me to let bygones be bygones. He said that I had had a wonderful career and I should let the past and the hate go.

As I say, I had so much time for Cyrille and so I agreed to try, but there was Paul, smiling and laughing. Smoke was coming out of my ears. The devil on my shoulder was laughing, saying there was no way I could let the past go, that I *was* going to go over there and let him have it. But I couldn't disrespect Cyrille, not him. He meant too much to me.

And then Paul came over. As he got closer, the devil's words were getting louder, but I couldn't lose it. Not there. Not now.

'Coley!' Elliott shouted. 'How's it going?'

No apology. Nothing. My eyes gave my rage away and immediately Elliott was on the defensive.

'Come on, Coley, it's not as if I saw any of that thirty grand.'

I couldn't believe it. No recognition that he might have called me, that someone should have spoken to me, a young footballer trying to make his way. Cyrille was there, so I couldn't go as mad as I wanted, but Elliott knew.

As I settled at Newcastle, I'd learnt just how murky football's waters could be, but also how cruel it is, as I never got a chance to say a proper goodbye to my team-mates, the staff or the fans in Bristol. That's life. I was now a Newcastle player and, with Clarky by my side, I got on with ingratiating myself with my new Geordie home.

Newcastle had a very good side. Kevin said to me that he'd signed me to get the team up, but that made me laugh because the squad had already been flying. They'd had a little blip in the new year and now, in March, it was time for the final push to the Premier League promised land. I certainly didn't expect to walk into the team.

Newcastle already had David 'Ned' Kelly and Gavin Peacock playing up front. Very good players. My first game was at a good Swindon side and I was on the bench. That was fine, but we lost 2–1 and I was straight in the team for the next game, at St James' Park against Notts County. Over 30,000 fans were there. A huge crowd for a First Division game at the time and proof that I was at a club very much on the up.

That itch that had formed while scoring reserve-team goals in front of a thousand fans at Arsenal had been gently scratched at Bristol City, playing in front of 10,000 people, but here, in front of such fanaticism and scoring my first goal in a 4–0 win, the scab was well and truly ripped off.

Clarky helped me settle, but so did the goals I scored. I knew the division well by now and I knew I could score in it, but mine had been a big move and, though I never worried about the fee, I knew eyebrows had

been raised by how much Kevin and his chairman, Sir
John Hall, had been prepared to pay.

I scored against Birmingham in a 2–2 draw that we'd
been losing 2–0. I scored at Cambridge and then I got
a hat-trick at home to Barnsley. I followed that up with
a late winner at Millwall. That win at the old Den was
massive and a game I relished in intimidating circumstances. Going to Millwall was always tricky, but I was
also facing Mick McCarthy, a big and tough centre-half.

Dropping down levels from Arsenal had put me up
against some tough defenders. When I was at Fulham,
I had faced Vince Overson and Noel Blake at Stoke.
Bloody hell, they were scary. I had never seen anything
like it. They would take turns coming through the back
of you. Physical? No, it was more like war. Tackles from
behind, the side, over the top. No prisoners were taken.

Painful as it could get, I relished it. Noel Blake was
huge. He had hands like shovels, but at the end of that
game, knowing that I had done OK and taken the abuse,
he came over to me. One of those big hands reached out
for my baby-looking one and he said, 'Well done, son.'
I knew then that I could handle the roughest of treatment.

At Millwall, McCarthy was just as combative, but by
now I'd got better. I was used to the intimidation, I was
ready for his rough stuff. I was also able to run Mick
all over the place. He hated that. He kept telling me
what he was going to do to me. He was funny, I'll give

him that. I actually liked him, but he wasn't happy with me. He couldn't keep up.

'I'm gonna break your leg, son.'

'Yeah, if you can catch me.'

It was up to the rest of the teams in the division to catch this Newcastle side, and it would prove an impossible task. I enjoyed being among the lads. Scott Sellars, Rob Lee, John Beresford, Steve Howey, Brian Kilcline, all proper players. Kilcline was a terrific guy. A big lion of a footballer but the most genuine man. The staff, too. Kevin, of course. His assistant, Terry McDermott, or the Barnet as we called him because of his fine head of hair. All were brilliant with me. I'd settled in and I felt the lads liked me.

At Arsenal I'd been liked, as I had in Bristol, but I wouldn't say it was vital to me. People can make up their minds quickly, of course. They always had done with me. I'm cocky, I'm arrogant. I was like Marmite at so many clubs that I went to. You either loved me or you hated me. No in between. For those who hated me, the 'arrogant' thing seemed to be the most common reason, but that just meant they hadn't taken the time – and it does take time – to get to know me.

Roy Keane at Manchester United used to say that you only need six real friends, because that's how many you need to carry a coffin. We used to laugh at how morbid he could be, but in football he's probably right.

I have met so many people in the game. Plenty haven't liked me and vice versa, but all you want is for that judgement to be a fair one.

At Newcastle, I felt at home. There were a few early issues with Paul Bracewell, one of the senior pros, but nothing too major. Brace was a great player and we'd be OK, but he could be a bit odd with the younger players. He had enjoyed a brilliant career with Everton, won loads, played for England, but it seemed strange to me that he would give the whole 'Show me your medals' line to young footballers who had only just started out on their career paths.

For now, we could show him our First Division Championship medals. The title was won at home to Oxford United in the season's penultimate game and was followed by a carnival 7–1 win at home to Leicester three days later. It was so special. A party-like atmosphere in front of a bouncing St James'. I scored the winner against Oxford to clinch the league and then got a hat-trick against Leicester.

I was going to be a Premier League footballer. I had gone my own way to get there, but I'd made it. Worries about whether or not I'd be able to continue scoring goals against the best defenders in the country were for another day. For now, I celebrated with my team-mates, with the management team and with the ecstatic fans who had immediately taken to me.

I celebrated with Kevin Keegan. Kevin and I had hit it off. He had filled me with confidence. He had persuaded his chairman to part with a lot of money for a young player with a bit of a bad-boy reputation and fewer than sixty games under his belt, and now we were going up to the top flight together to test ourselves. All I could think was, bring it on.

In that close season, Kevin took me to one side. 'There's going to be a few changes,' he said.

'OK,' I replied, slightly confused about what he meant. I mean I was just a player in a very good squad.

'I'm moving a few on.'

'OK, boss.' It was a bit awkward because the lads were my mates and I didn't want to know too much.

'I'm selling David Kelly.'

I was shocked. Ned was a top pro. He'd played top-flight football and was one of the most honest players around. Kevin himself used to say he'd chase a piece of paper.

'Why are you moving Ned on?' I asked. 'He's a great player.'

'Not good enough for where we're going, son.' He had a twinkle in his eye. 'Don't worry, though, Coley. I've got someone lined up, and he's just for you.'

5

NOTHING IS BLACK AND WHITE

I'd found centre-forward nirvana. A football team built to accommodate my game. A midfield able to keep things ticking over, able to win possession, keep it, get the ball wide, able to find a pass. Footballers with a feel for the game. Paul Bracewell in midfield, anchoring, tidy. Lee Clark, dynamic, always looking forward, the proudest of Geordies, willing to give his last breath to the team. Rob Lee, a fantastic player, a mixture of graft and creativity. Scott Sellars, a wand of a left foot, able to find me effortlessly time and time again.

None had real pace, but what a group of footballers. With my pace up front, the team had a good balance, but good wasn't good enough. Not for what our manager had in mind. Good was mid-table. Kevin Keegan was aiming for the stars and for that he needed more, and more came in the shape of Peter Beardsley.

Going into the Premier League didn't worry me. I'm not fazed by the unknown. I embrace it. I love a challenge.

I was looking forward to it, the whole club was, but to be honest, after we won the First Division, glancing around the dressing room and the faces in it, there wasn't a lot of top-flight experience.

Barry Venison, Bracewell, Brian Kilcline, Rob Lee? The rest of us were stepping into the unknown, but then along came Peter Beardsley, a shining beacon of talent and experience. Peter had been the player that Kevin, like an excited dad on Christmas Eve, had promised me. I couldn't have asked for a better present.

Peter was perfect for my game. He would link with those other guys, beat a man, play me or someone else in. Talk about football intelligence. Peter's IQ was off the charts. Modern footballing jargon like 'Playing between the lines' sounds fancy and new, doesn't it? Peter was doing that in the 1980s and 1990s.

In football, space is like gold. In the Premier League, it's platinum. Peter had a way of finding it and exploiting it. He'd drop into pockets, drop a shoulder, beat a man, and with a simple but brilliant pass I was in.

You couldn't help but learn from him. I had pace, I made runs in behind high lines of defence, but Peter had different ways of looking at the game. 'Stand still,' he once said to me. I'd never heard that before. I had been coached to run into space, to seek it out. Peter had this knack of doing things differently. 'You don't always have to run. Let them do the running. Check, stop and let the space find you.'

If you watch old footage of Peter, that's exactly what he would do. Look at the goalscorers his game benefited. Kevin Keegan himself at Newcastle, John Aldridge and Ian Rush at Liverpool, Gary Lineker with England. All of them very different players, but so good was Peter at adapting, and so clever was his game, all of them filled their boots with goals.

Kevin had me on top of his Christmas tree. The players behind me could battle, pass and, boom, a spark from Peter and I was in. And in. And in again. The 1993–94 season saw me score forty-one goals in all competitions, thirty-four in the Premier League.

I couldn't have dreamt of it going any better. Playing in this brilliant side, scoring goal after goal in front of the adoring Geordies who came to St James' Park – and every other ground where we played – in their thousands. The joy in their faces, the atmosphere they created, it was the most exciting ride, and driving us all the way was the manager, Kevin Keegan.

Kevin was more than a hero in Newcastle. Charismatic and energetic, that's how he wanted his team to be. Small in stature, Kevin got right to the top of the game, winning everything. In Germany they called him Mighty Mouse, and you could tell he saw his team, small in terms of recent history but – with his enthusiasm and with the most passionate fans in the country roaring us on – capable of being the mightiest around.

Kevin understood Geordies. He knew what could be achieved with them behind us. It's not enough to simply have passionate fans, though; you need a manager who knows exactly how to light a fire under that passion. Kevin was that man.

He was very much influenced by his time at Liverpool. He was modern and could also draw on his time in Germany, but his days at Anfield were clearly the biggest influence. Years later I worked with Graeme Souness, who wouldn't stop talking about Bob Paisley and Joe Fagan, and Kevin had the same admiration for Bill Shankly. His teams needed to get it, pass it and move, and as with Shankly, the relationship between supporters and the team was vital to any success.

Kevin's Liverpool links stretched to his choice of assistant. The Barnet was funny. I liked him. We used to give him loads of stick. Terry never said much in work, he just left Kevin to do all the talking. They were best mates and we'd make jokes about jobs for the boys.

Terry was so unassuming. On away trips he'd get the sandwiches, and we'd be giving him loads. 'Three-time European Cup winner, fetching the sandwiches!' He always took it well and, in all honesty, you couldn't do anything but respect Terry. The things he had achieved in the game and the quality player he was, you had to respect him. We all liked him a lot.

Also popular on Keegan's staff was first-team coach Derek Fazackerley. I say popular, but Faz was in charge of pre-season training, and he was very far from being my favourite person that summer we prepared for life in the Premier League.

I was never a fan of pre-season. Not my cup of tea at all. But in the summer of 1993 I was actually looking forward to it, looking forward to getting strong. Back then, players had a proper off-season. Six to eight weeks. We would relax, go away with mates, get unfit. Pre-season would hurt, but this time, being a Premier League footballer, I was raring to go.

Ten minutes into the first day back, and I realised why I hated pre-season. Faz and Terry Mac had us running hills through the forest at Maiden Castle in Durham, and it was painful. I hated it so much. Hills and mud. It was so tiring. I was too tired to puke. No, even in those exciting days, pre-season wasn't for me.

It wasn't long before the lads and staff at Newcastle gathered that I wasn't a big fan of giving everything in training. Kevin was on me, always on me. That wasn't a problem. Kevin's whole game had been about his natural enthusiasm, and he expected the same from his players. Give it your all, always. There were plenty in the squad who did just that.

Venners was one. He was crazy. As loud as his jackets. He was always 110 per cent. Never stopped. I think he was a bit hyperactive. He lived fast. Always on the go. That just isn't me, and he'd be on at me in training. 'Come on, Coley, give more!' Brace was the same, and John Beresford. Bez even went to Kevin complaining about me. I liked Bez, and didn't begrudge him doing that. I just didn't understand them.

'Train like you play' was the line. That idea defeats me. Why do that? If you train like you play, every day, then what will you have left on the Saturday? That's the most important thing to me: the match. For me, training was all about ticking over, doing what I had to do to be ready for the weekend. If I had trained like those guys, I'd have been a waste of time come match day. Simple as that.

I could understand my team-mates' issues. There they were, knocking their pipes out, looking at me, and in their eyes, I was strolling. There were frustrations. Kevin himself would get in my ear. 'Andrew, you have to train like the rest,' he'd say. 'Look, you can take time off, but you have to put in a shift like the others.' I'd smile, nod and say, 'Yes, boss,' but it was never for me. It wasn't a big problem between us. In fact, I think he understood me, but his own natural enthusiasm couldn't stop him having a gentle moan.

It had been my 'attitude' that actually appealed to

Kevin when he was thinking about signing me. He and the Barnet came to see me at Ashton Gate. I had damaged my knee. Ligaments, I think. I played anyway and got out there heavily bandaged. My form and goals were one thing, but the fact that I had gone out there and played through the pain, that was enough for Kevin. He'd seen my own kind of natural enthusiasm on show.

Kevin and I were good. What I didn't show in training, I showed at the weekend. I was hungry for goals and he could see that. He liked it. I liked him. He had this irresistible positivity. Before the season kicked off he was setting targets – and they were lofty. Usually when a team comes into the Premier League for the first time, it's all about consolidation. Conservative targets. Just stay up, find your feet. That's not Kevin, though. He was talking top four, maybe higher.

I was thinking, hold on, hardly any of us have played at this level before, but to Kevin none of that mattered. He was sure we could be right up there, and eventually it was infectious. He would talk so enthusiastically about just going out there and enjoying ourselves and I began to think, why not?

Such lofty optimism took a hit just days before the season started when Peter Beardsley, in a friendly at Liverpool, fractured his jaw. Well, he had his jaw fractured for him. Neil Ruddock. It was a naughty challenge. Totally unnecessary from a player just trying to live up to his hard-man tag. It was a big blow. We were about to take our first steps into the big league, and now, without our best player, those steps were far more tentative.

So tentative that we lost our first two games. Tottenham beat us at St James' and then we lost at Coventry. The defeats underlined the team's weaknesses at the back. Without Peter, we lacked that spark, and we would struggle to be compact. We leaked goals.

Our offensive style was a ballsy approach, especially in the Premier League. In defence we had good players. In goal there was Pavel Srnicek. He was a great lad, Pav, God rest his soul. He could make a worldy save one minute and the ball was going through his legs the next. He was very popular and, on his day, brilliant. 'Pavel is a Geordie,' the fans would sing. He loved that.

Kevin also signed Mike Hooper from Liverpool. For half a million. That was a strange one for me. For all of Pav's odd mistakes, I didn't think Mike was any better than him. Mike was carrying a bit of weight and he would make plenty of ricks. I think Kevin was confused about who to play out of the two and it was unsettling.

Whoever did play, they had good footballers in front of them. Venners was a fantastic player. He had a real

Indian summer at Newcastle, getting into the England team. He was versatile and would play across the back-line and sometimes in midfield. At the centre of our defence was Steve Howey and Kevin Scott. Steve was really good. He could have had some career but for bad luck and injuries. Kevin was a local lad, solid, but he left for Tottenham that season. Steve Watson was coming through and John Beresford was a great pro.

Darren Peacock joined us later in the season and was good in the air, but it was the later signing of the defender Philippe Albert that brought real quality. Philippe, my God, he was some footballer. I'm not overstating it when I say Philippe could have been up there with the very best. He was quality. What a left foot he had. He wanted to play. He'd step out with the ball, carry it forward, look to play one-twos. The thing that held Philippe back was his lack of understanding of the English game.

I think the physicality of the game here shocked Philippe. He wanted to play but he didn't like the rough stuff. If a striker started leaving it on him, Philippe was like, 'Nah, that's not for me. I'm not having this.' He was a big man, great in the air, but it was that side of the game that he didn't take to and forwards exploited it. You can't teach a player to be nasty. I'm sure Philippe had the talent to play for any club in the world, though, and he's certainly one of the best I ever played with.

Marc Hottiger would also join, at right-back. A Swiss international, Marc was a really nice kid. Like the team as a whole, Marc was ridiculous going forward, less good at defending. You got the feeling that that didn't bother Kevin. A manager hell-bent on attack. That's where Kevin's priorities lay. 'What about when they have the ball?' we'd ask, but Kevin's philosophy was simply 'We'll cause them more problems than they cause us.'

This, though, was the Premier League, and those two early defeats – albeit without Peter – had some onlookers wondering if we were ready to be there. Defeats at Newcastle always left a cloud over the place. Kevin was so emotional. Maybe too emotional. He would get very low, a proper monk on for days, and it would bring the whole place down.

Venners used to hate it. He didn't like people moping about and the manager's moods used to get to him. They'd row like a married couple. The thing is, come the Thursday, Kevin would be back on a high. 'Come on then, lads, let's go! Match on Saturday!' We'd be like, 'Hold on, what about the mood?' Suddenly you had to start skipping to his beat again. I found it hard, too.

Our third game that season was at Old Trafford. Manchester United were the new champions and a third straight defeat was on the cards, and who knows what

that would do to our, or more importantly our manager's, morale. Kevin had us all on it that day and we
played well. Ryan Giggs put them one up, but in the
second half we were very good, and I managed to get
away from Steve Bruce and finish neatly past Peter
Schmeichel to get us a more than decent draw.

From there, we found our feet. Peter came back from
his injury and we put a good run of results together.
When it came to my home life, though, I was finding
it harder to settle in. After I signed, without an agent
to offer decent advice, I had got myself a place in a
small mining town called Crook. Kevin thought it was
best that I live near the training ground. It was only
twenty minutes away, so that was bang on, but this was
in the middle of nowhere, a small place, full of lovely
people but with absolutely nothing to do.

My house was in a little close, and my neighbours
were all very nice, but they wouldn't leave me alone.
Every half-hour there would be a knock on my door.

'Would you like some milk?' one neighbour would
ask.

'No, thank you, I'm fine.'

Half an hour later, the door would go again.

'We've baked you a cake. Would you like it?'

'Thank you, but I'm fine.'

And on and on.

I would go to London for a few days, come back late at night and straight away there would be a knock on the door. 'The house is fine.' It makes me smile, looking back and thinking how nice those people were, but at the time being cut off was frustrating me and I felt lonely. Eventually, I moved to a hotel, before getting an apartment in the city itself.

With Newcastle's black and white stripes on my back, I had no problem feeling at home. After the Manchester United game, we went on a seven-game unbeaten run and I got seven goals. And then there was a problem.

It was October 1993, but I remember it like it was yesterday. We'd travelled down for the weekend's game to Southampton. It was coach travel back then. A long and tiring journey and I was feeling it. We had lost 2–1 at the Dell. I'd scored our goal but I walked off that pitch with heavy legs and a heavier mind.

It was a hard day. We'd not played well and the dressing room was tense. Clarky had been subbed towards the end of the game and wasn't happy. Clarky was a mad competitor and, being a Geordie, he hated both losing and being taken off. He wasn't having it and instead of joining the bench, he went for the dressing room.

At Southampton's old Dell stadium, the dressing rooms were in the corner of the pitch, so it would have been a bit of a walk for him, but before he really got going, Kevin had him by his collar and was dragging him back to the bench. It didn't look good. You can't make Clarky look like some naughty kid, not Clarky, a player who always gives everything.

I was hacked off. Clarky had become my best mate and if you treat my best mate like that, I'm not going to be happy. It was a tense dressing room and the bad atmosphere just added to my feelings of frustration and fatigue. It would get worse.

Our next game was just three days later, a League Cup tie at Wimbledon, and so instead of heading back to Newcastle, we drove up to Selsdon Park, a hotel near Croydon, south London. We had the Sunday off but trained nearby on the Monday, and the fatigue I had felt all weekend was still there. Things were affecting me. The travel, the long distances, the games. It was all slowing me down, and the manager could see it.

'Coley!' Kevin shouted from the touchline. 'What's wrong? Do you not fancy it today?' It was a simple question and I gave a simple answer.

'I'm tired, boss,' I said.

'Well, if you don't fancy it, then **** off.'

I couldn't believe it. The words hung in the air, stopping me in my tracks. Things had been getting on top of me. I'd worked hard, scored goals. I was tired and I was honest about it. But there it was: '**** off.' It bubbled and it bubbled. I had had enough. I walked off the pitch.

I was thinking to myself, 'You don't understand me.' Kevin and I had never had cross words before, but there it was, and I was telling myself, 'This guy has no idea where I'm coming from.' If someone says that to me, especially back then, I immediately think, 'Well **** you too.' That's how I'd reacted when Pat Rice had said something similar at Arsenal. Nothing had changed. My mum had always taught me to speak my mind, and so, if someone had come at me in that aggressive manner, effing and blinding, they'd better expect it back.

I got showered, dressed, packed my bag and I left, thinking, 'Stuff football. I'm off.'

Shirley was living in Brixton at the time, not far away, so I got myself there and arrived at her door, unannounced.

'What are you doing here?' she said as I made my way in.

'I just fell out with the manager.'

'Why do you always do that?' she asked. 'Why do you always react? Why do you always lose it and walk out?'

I could hear her but her words made no difference. My mind was made up. I switched my phone off and stayed quietly at hers. I was genuinely ready to jack it in. I was in love with football, but what people didn't understand was that if you talk to me in a certain way, in the way Kevin did, you have to be prepared for me to react, and react hard.

Shirley couldn't understand that. Why was I jeopardising my career? Maybe she was right, but back then I wasn't going to change. I wasn't going to back down. We all come from different places, different backgrounds, and deal with things in our own way. I wasn't going to accept it. Not from Kevin. Not from anyone.

The situation was made worse by the team's 2–1 defeat at Wimbledon, but for me the touchpaper was lit when it became clear that someone at the club had briefed the press. ANDY GOES AWOL was all over the back pages. Wow. I was furious. Here we go, my attitude called into question again. No questions asked, just taken as read.

I was adamant that the problem hadn't been caused by me. I had been honest, I had addressed the fact that I was feeling tired, and I had been told to **** off. That was the problem. Simple as. Today, player fatigue is addressed by coaches; sports scientists gauge it, monitor it; players are looked after. I tell my manager that I'm tired and I'm told to **** off. What a load of nonsense.

By now I had got myself an agent, Paul Stretford,

and soon he was on the phone. 'You have to go back,' he said. I wasn't going to back down, but I knew I had to be seen sooner rather than later and so I went for a meeting with Kevin and the Barnet, my agent and Freddy Shepherd, the Newcastle director. We all sat in Shep's living room, and I got to say my piece. We agreed to move on, but from that moment, things between Kevin and me were never the same. Like a failed relationship, the romance had gone.

The goals wouldn't stop, though. Whatever our newly formed problems, Kevin put me straight back into the team and I continued to find the net. I was being talked about as a top goalscorer and it felt good. It was a feeling that only got better one freezing November Sunday afternoon when Liverpool came to St James' in front of the Sky Sports cameras.

We absolutely blitzed them. Liverpool were struggling towards the end of Graeme Souness's time as manager there, but they were still one of the Premier League's big hitters, and the way we took them apart, it felt like the moment we'd arrived. We could have been six up before half-time, but we settled for three. I got the first after just four minutes, my second ten minutes later and my hat-trick on the half-hour.

We were buzzing all round them. All the goals came

from attacking their left. I was a bit gutted not to add my own or the team's tally in the second half, but the damage had been done and the game won. Later, it was said that their keeper, Bruce Grobbelaar, had thrown the goals in as part of his alleged match-fixing, but I'm not having that. They could have had two keepers that day and I would have scored.

My confidence was that high. I expected to score, I was getting goals and the team were climbing the league. Soon, I was the talk of the Toon. The No. 9 shirt that meant so much to the club and its followers had a new owner, and in the north-east that was massive. To be honest, things like squad numbers didn't really bother me. I could wear any shirt and would have backed myself to score. When I arrived at Newcastle I wore the No. 8, and that was fine by me. After we got promoted Kevin came to me and said he wanted me to take the No. 9. It didn't seem a big deal to me – I was happy enough with No. 8 – but Kevin was adamant.

He explained the significance of the shirt, what it meant to the fans. Kevin wanted the team to have even more of a connection with the punters. Peter Beardsley was in my ear about it too, so all right, I'll take it. I didn't feel any extra weight with the number on my back. I was too busy enjoying myself to let it get to me. As I say, I would have taken any number, and let's not forget that plenty of Newcastle No. 9s had stunk too. It wasn't a magic number. I knew I had to work to get my goals, that was the important thing, and that's just what I did.

Soon, my name was being talked about in the same breath as one of the all-time Newcastle greats. Hughie Gallacher had scored thirty-nine goals in all competitions in the 1926–27 seasons, and with each goal I got, talk became louder about the chances of me getting more. Records didn't really matter to me, but when Douglas Hall, Sir John's son, said that if I beat it, he'd get me a BMW M3, I started to take a little more notice.

Douglas and I got on. We were always joking together and he'd say things like 'If you get a hat-trick on Saturday, I'll pay for you to have a posh weekend in London,' or 'I'll get you a suit.' He'd say, 'Get two goals this week and you can have a Versace tie.' I'd score the goals and he'd give me the tie from around his own neck.

The players found out about it and it didn't go down well at all, especially when they heard about the record and the BMW. It was just a bit of fun, but my teammates didn't like the idea that I was getting a few extras, and nor did Kevin. It was just a laugh between two mates, but the manager was worried about team morale.

*

When it came to morale, expensive gifts were one thing, but goals and wins were another, and with the team flying high in the league and me just one goal behind Gallacher's record, the atmosphere at St James' on an April evening was electric. Over 32,000 bouncing Geordies and when, five minutes before half-time, I raced clear and not only put us 3–1 up against Aston Villa but broke Gallacher's record, the place went nuts.

It was my fortieth goal of an incredible season. I had proved some people wrong, but I had also changed a few old perceptions. Newcastle and the north-east hadn't had much history with black footballers but now they were hero-worshipping one.

Tony Cunningham, a Jamaican striker, had played a couple of seasons in the 1980s. It was a decade when the nickname 'Blackie Milburn', given to him from the terraces, was thought acceptable and so there were barriers that needed to be broken down. I can look back at my time up there with great positivity because I helped do just that.

The key, though, was doing well. No disrespect to Cunningham, but if I'd not scored I'd have been forgotten and old perceptions can remain. It's mad, but it takes success to change people's views on things and my goals helped. Ruel Fox joined us that season and Foxy said that me being there and doing well had made him feel comfortable about making the move. Les Ferdinand would later tell me the same thing.

Football has the ability to show bigots that it isn't the colour of a man's skin that defines him. I went to Newcastle, hit the ground running and quickly changed how some people thought about things. Early on in my time there, my brother and a couple of friends were racially abused walking from the ground to their car. That disappointed me, but no one ever said anything to me that could be called abusive.

Actually, the people couldn't have been nicer. They had so much time for me and were so friendly, but the intensity of the place, with Newcastle being a one-club city, it got well on top. I've mentioned that I was never in football for the adulation and I never courted fame. I am like a punter playing – I love the game, I want the glory, I want to see the team win – but in Newcastle, I'd be lying if I said I enjoyed the attention that came with my success.

I loved making them happy on a Saturday, scoring, taking the applause, seeing the people leave with a smile on their face, but then I wanted to chill, take a breath, have my downtime. In Newcastle, I'd sometimes go out for dinner on a Saturday and people would come and want to talk, get an autograph. I found that hard.

I was once in a supermarket doing a weekly shop and got swamped by people. I couldn't handle it. I had to get away and just left a full trolley in the aisle, so I could get to my car. I could have done with online shopping being invented back then, because my home became my haven, the place where I could chill, where I could switch off.

People could see I struggled with all that and they made up their minds that I was stand-offish, that I was this arrogant footballer who had no time for the fans who paid my wages. That wasn't true at all. I wanted to make their lives happier by scoring goals and helping their beloved team to win. But, after the game, I needed to have downtime. I wasn't aloof, I wasn't rude, I am just very private.

In that, I was the complete opposite of Kevin. Kevin loved the limelight. He was one of football's first super-stars and while he never let it get in the way of the hard work he always put into his game, you knew he loved what he got from his public. After his last game as a Newcastle player, he had left the pitch and his adoring people in a helicopter. In me, I'm sure the fans saw someone less able to give them what they wanted, and away from the pitch they found it harder to take to me.

I'm not knocking the Geordies at all. They were brilliant. It's the fame in general that I, still a very young man, struggled with. The bit I loved was the football, and that was going better than I could have dreamt.

The last game of the season was against my old team, Arsenal, and I was desperate to score against them and rub my success in a few people's faces.

I scored in a 2–0 win. Have a bit of humble pie, I thought. We finished third, capping off a brilliant first season back in the top flight, and I won the Premier League's Golden Boot and was named the PFA's Young Player of the Year. That summer I was buzzing. I had made it. I was good enough not only to play at this level but to excel at it.

My relationship with Kevin might have cooled off, but that's football, I could live with that, and the team were doing great. I was just happy for my family. They could all see that the hard work that had gone into getting me there was worth it. As long as they were proud, I was happy. Life was great at Newcastle, but who knew what was just around the corner?

6

HEAVEN SENT

The cold January night moves by the car window. My agent, Paul, is driving us from Newcastle to Manchester and we sit in silence. My thoughts are elsewhere. The distant Pennines blur into the dark sky, matching my confused and bleak mood.

I'm about to become a Manchester United player. A childhood dream, but the nature of football has soured the moment. The story will soon break and as I look out onto the M62, I know how it will play out. I can see the headlines before they've been written:

'COLE FORCES MOVE TO MANCHESTER UNITED'
'COLE TURNS HIS BACK ON ADORING GEORDIES'

I've been mugged off. For so long, people have carried those perceptions of me. They've questioned my attitude, my ability, they've decided quickly about my character, and now they will make up their minds about this. I am going to be the bad guy here, the spoilt footballer wanting more, deserting the hand that feeds him.

As we approach the city, just ahead of us we can see

the Manchester United team bus. They are almost home after winning at Sheffield United. The lads will be laughing, sharing a joke, and as we overtake them I think about how surreal life can be, how fast things can change. On the bus are a group of footballers who tomorrow I will call team-mates, but they don't know that, hardly anyone knows. Very soon they will.

As 1994 turned into 1995, footballers were becoming the news. Magazines such as *Loaded* had Premier League faces on their covers, party invites dropped through players' letter boxes and onto their marble floors. Footballers from abroad were eyeing up our game and dusting off their passports. Glamorous celebrities wanted to be seen on the arms of footballers, and the world watched.

With our new-found fame came other people's opinions. The public was making up its mind about us. We were becoming seen as spoilt, overpaid prima donnas, and as the league's top scorer I was going to be judged. Each of the forty-one goals I had scored in the 1993–94 season had hurtled me into the public consciousness and now news of my move to Manchester United would be met with assumption rather than fact. *He's got here, we've given him his chance and his success, now he's off, leaving us for a bigger club.* These would be the

initial thoughts of those Newcastle fans who had idolised me only days before.

In his recent autobiography, even Kevin Keegan
himself suggested that his gut feeling was that I had
been tapped up back in 1995 and that I had looked for
the move to Manchester United. That is total nonsense.
I was happy at Newcastle. I was settling into the city
and life as footballer. Yes, Kevin and I were no longer
as close as we had been, but that wasn't a big deal to
me. I was learning my trade there. I was still only young.
I never presumed to think I'd made it, that the season
I had and all the goals I had scored meant I was the
finished article. I felt I was in the right place at Newcastle
and thoughts of leaving just weren't there.

I've talked about how well Kevin and I had got on
when I first arrived at Newcastle. We had a connection.
I felt the team was built for me. Peter Beardsley had
been bought for me. I'm not being big-headed when I
say that, but Kevin would treat me like the cherry on
top of his cake.

One afternoon in the previous season I had arrived
at St James' to pick up some mail.

'Coley, what are you up to?' Kevin shouted from his
office.

'Nothing, boss, just getting my post.'

'You got a coat?'

'No.'

'That doesn't matter, we have plenty here. Grab one. You're coming to Anfield with me.'

Together we drove to watch Liverpool play Queens Park Rangers. He'd ask me what I thought of Les Ferdinand, how we could play together. He asked about other players and shortly afterwards the club signed Darren Peacock, whose name had come up in our discussion that night.

The incident in training that had made me walk out on the club had changed things, but I, like Kevin, went into the 1994–95 season buzzing, wanting to do well, maybe go even higher than third in the Premier League, maybe win a trophy, test ourselves in Europe. I don't know if he found it hard to manage me. I did things my way a lot, but in my defence I was also a great self-manager.

I had a burning desire and passion to achieve as much as possible. I might have preferred to go about it the way I thought best, but I wanted to get there as much as any manager. My internal observations were intense. I didn't need managers and coaches telling me I was in the wrong or I hadn't played well, because I already knew. I'd already had that conversation. Maybe that's why I didn't respond to criticism the way people expected or wanted me to.

Whatever differences there now were between Kevin and me, I was desperate to prove all over again that I was here to stay. I had scored forty-one goals but, this being football, people were waiting to label me 'a one-season wonder'. In football you have to enjoy the sunshine while you can, because people will always enjoy knocking you down. I was a marked man, defenders often doubling up on me, but I was scoring.

Getting forty-one goals was never going to happen again, but I was comfortable, in a good team and looking forward. We were unbeaten in our first eleven Premier League games. I scored eight goals. We beat Chelsea, won at Arsenal, got a point off a rejuvenated Liverpool and high-flying Blackburn. We won at West Ham and at Villa. Things were good.

We'd eventually get beaten at Old Trafford, but we were challenging at the top of the ever-growing Premier League. Newcastle United were going places. I was loving my football. I loved the challenges the league threw up. The defenders I was facing were the elite, all offering a different way of thinking.

Facing Manchester United, that was hard. Steve Bruce and Gary Pallister – I'd say the best partnership around. Steve was a brilliant footballer. Strong, clever, he might have lacked pace but no one ever ran him, because he was on top of you. No England caps? I really don't get that.

Pally was his opposite. Whereas Bruce would come through you and beat you with force, Pally would try to nick the ball away from you, stretch in front of you and steal possession from you. I'd get to know both well, very soon.

At Blackburn there was Colin Hendry. He was a competitor. Some called him 'Mr Braveheart', but we used to call him 'Mr Last Ditch'. He'd always be on the stretch, sliding in at the last minute. Great player.

Chris Fairclough at Leeds was quick and strong; so was his team-mate John Pemberton. I loved facing quick central defenders. Tony and Bouldy at Arsenal were always letting you know, never afraid of leaving one in – just like they'd been in training. Paul McGrath at Villa was special. Later, Dwight Yorke used to tell me just how good he was. He wouldn't train through the week because of his knees, but every Saturday he was the outstanding player in the team. Hands down.

Des Walker was a favourite of mine. Before I left home, us kids in Nottingham would have a game and Des, who was at Forest, would come and join in. He wasn't allowed – this was one of the best defenders in Europe – but he'd get involved. I used to say to myself, 'I want to play against him properly one day.'

Then I did. He was at Sheffield Wednesday by that stage and I used to love the battles against him. He was rapid. The race was always on. He was brilliant at trying to steer you into the corners and we'd have a laugh. 'You've come a long way,' he said to me when we first met again. A phenomenal footballer.

Sol Campbell was brilliant at Tottenham. Sol loved it. Always in your ear, giving it the verbals. I didn't mind all that. Some of it was quite funny. It could get nasty but I would ignore it. I'd played in the second and third tiers, where defenders didn't mess about. Players like Ian Wright might blow up, but the verbals never bothered me. Well, hardly ever. The only one that got in my head was Keith Curle at Manchester City.

I'd have running battles with him. Take nothing away from him, he was quick, but we would have words. He was always telling me this and that. He relied too much on his pace, though, and I could get the better of him. I couldn't put my finger on what it was about Keith, but he got into my head and I took pleasure scoring against him.

As autumn turned to winter I had a small goal drought. That didn't bother me, we all have them, but what I didn't realise was that Kevin was starting to have his doubts about me, wondering if I'd lost my edge. He even dropped me. Again, that didn't bother me, it happens, and I was soon back in the team. The club had even given me a new contract.

I've mentioned that by now I had an agent. I had been introduced to Paul Stretford the season before. I had left Crook by then, and moved into a hotel. Scott

Sellars was there too and he suggested that if it was some advice I needed, then I should meet his agent. 'He'll be good for you.'

I thought about it and agreed to meet him and Paul was all smooth talk. It went in one ear and out the other because I'd heard all the same stuff from Steve Waggott.

'What that other guy done, I would never do that,' Paul said.

Paul said I could sign with him for one year, and if I didn't fancy it, I could cancel the agreement. Why not? I had a contract, that was done, so what was there to lose? There were smaller things to sort, boot deals maybe, and it would be good to get decent advice about things. So I signed.

Newcastle had come to me with a new contract after my goal-scoring feats in my debut Premier League campaign. It was a good deal, right up there with the senior pros, but I think that upset some of them. There was a bit of animosity; players were put out that this young striker was getting as much as them, if not more.

Then I had a bad Christmas. I hadn't scored, and after a FA Cup third round draw at home to Blackburn, we trained on Monday. Kevin was quiet but that was normal. We hadn't played well. I went home, preparing to watch Manchester United take on Sheffield United on the telly later that evening. And then I got a phone call. It was Paul Stretford.

'Coley, you know you once said that you'd only leave Newcastle for Manchester United?'

'Yes.'

'Well, the deal's on.'

Paul was right, I had recently said just that to him. In the summer of 1994, Ossie Ardiles, the Tottenham manager, had made a £5 million bid for me, one which I had quickly rejected even before Newcastle had had their say. 'Only Manchester United would get me away,' I'd said, but it was a flippant comment. It couldn't really happen.

'No.' That was my first reaction. 'No, it isn't. There's no way that's true, Paul,' I said. I just didn't believe that Kevin would agree to it. I didn't believe that Alex Ferguson would even try it.

'What about my new contract?' I asked.

'It's done, Andrew. Kevin has decided that the £6 million United have offered, plus Keith Gillespie coming the other way, is too good to turn down.'

I was stunned. I felt that, despite our differences, Kevin and I could work together. I'd gone those few games without a goal, but I'd still got fifteen that season and plenty more would follow in the black and white of Newcastle. Only, now they wouldn't.

'It's done, Coley. The deal's done.'

With those words in my ears, Paul picked me up and we headed to Manchester that night, and as we drove, I sat quietly, uncomfortable with what had just happened. A phone call broke the silence. It was Kevin.

'I think the deal's right for you, Andy,' he started. 'It's Manchester United. A fantastic club. You'll learn even more there, you'll win things there, the time is right. We've got good money, Keith is a promising young player. Good luck, mate.'

It was brutal and it hurt. It didn't sit well with me. Why now? Why had they just given me a lucrative contract? And there were those concerns about the public's perceptions. I knew what the narrative would be. I hadn't forced anything, but the fans would believe, for years, that it was me who had manipulated the situation, that it was me who wanted away. As I've said, that is simply not true. Maybe their love for Kevin made it easier for them to think I was the bad guy, I don't know, but there was that negativity around me again.

What I didn't like was the lack of control. No one had talked to me. The fans weren't happy and hundreds of them descended on the stadium to protest. I should have been touched, but there was Kevin, able to come out and argue his case. It was typical of Kevin. Brilliant. He was a showman. He understood the power he had, he understood how the fans felt.

Kevin stood there on those steps. A messiah. While he explained that it was his final decision to sell, it wasn't made clear that I had absolutely no part in securing the move. 'Andy forced it' was still what the fans thought had happened, and though Kevin was able to get up and say his bit, I wasn't.

Oh well, I had a new life to get used to. I was a Manchester United player.

It was hard to take in. My mate Paul Ince at United had always joked with me. 'The gaffer likes you,' he'd say. 'He wants you to join us.'

'No chance,' I'd always said. It had seemed so far-fetched, but here I was, the following day, walking into a new training ground, meeting new team-mates, players that only hours before I'd considered rivals.

I was overawed. This was Manchester United. The players welcoming me were the best around. Huge names. Schmeichel, Pallister, Bruce, Keane, Ince, Irwin, Hughes, Cantona. I had only been in the Premier League a season and a half. It wasn't long ago that I was at Bristol City. I was a kid. Won nothing. Here I was in the biggest dressing room in the country. Did I have a right to be there?

Luckily the players seemed to think I did. 'Thank God I don't have to chase you about any more,' Steve

Bruce said, immediately putting me at ease. There would be a problem, though. I had no boots. The move had happened so quickly, nothing had come with me. As with Bristol City, not even a chance to say goodbye. That's football.

For ages, Kevin had been on at me to buy a place in the north-east, to settle down, and finally I had. A lovely new apartment in the town centre. I'd had it all kitted out, it was smart. Now, having only just moved in, I was off. I ended up renting it to Les Ferdinand. For the record, he was a very good tenant.

My new landlord was Alex Ferguson. For all the uncertainty I had felt driving to Manchester, one meeting with him and I knew this was right for me. I've talked about the false perceptions people too often had of me. Well, I'll admit that I had my own ideas of the gaffer. Gruff, hard to please, tough. You hear things from other people, but then you meet him and you realise what an incredible man he is.

He has this aura, this way of talking to you about the club and the game. I don't think many footballers who met Ferguson to discuss a possible move didn't end up signing. I was sold. Having sat down and talked, I wasn't even interested in the numbers. Wages would look after themselves. I just wanted to get started. But why me?

The boss told me that he had looked at Stan

Collymore, too, but what he liked about me was how nimble I was, how my movement suited the team. I later heard that Stan was furious when he found out Manchester United had signed me over him, even walking out of the training ground at Nottingham Forest, but I was happy to hear a man of the gaffer's stature saying that I was a player his great team needed.

United, he said, were now playing against more defensive sides, teams that would crowd the penalty box, and he needed a striker who could get it into his feet, turn quickly, get shots away in tight spaces, and that he liked my hunger to get in behind. Mark Hughes was a physical presence and Eric was Eric, but I offered what he wanted. When do I start?

Brian Kidd, the manager's assistant, also had a word with me and made me realise exactly where I now worked. Kiddo congratulated me on the forty-one goals I had scored the previous season, but then said that wouldn't be enough here. He didn't mean that I needed to score forty-two. He meant that being a Manchester United player was about so much more. He meant that I had to carry myself in a certain way, that the team was everything and that just focusing on goals wouldn't do. He'd played under Sir Matt Busby, and so Kiddo knew.

*

That's why what happened in only my second game was such a shock to me. We were at Crystal Palace. Eric had an altercation with Richard Shaw and was sent off. As he walked to the tunnel along the side of the pitch, from the corner of my eye I saw a blur of movement. Eric had attacked an abusive fan. I did a double-take. What had just happened?

From there, I was in pure shock. Eric was a one-off and so his actions didn't completely shock me, but this was Manchester United. Things like that didn't happen at this football club. Everything was done with military precision. Suits on, shirts pressed, shoes polished, time-keeping spot on or else. But what had I just seen? I was stunned.

After drawing the game, we went into the dressing room and Eric was dressed and sitting quietly. No one said anything. The boss walked in and piled into Pally and David May, the centre-half. We were all thinking, 'Really?' He then turned to Eric and calmly said, 'Eric, you can't do things like that.' That was that.

That became the norm. Ferguson understood how to handle a personality like Eric. Us players would have a laugh about it, because despite all the bollockings given out by the boss, and the reputation he – rightly – had for letting a slack footballer know who was the boss, Eric never got any of it.

Once, the whole squad was invited to a film premiere

in Manchester. It was a nice bit of fun, but being Manchester United, the players had strict instructions about what to wear. Black tie. So, there we all were at the cinema in our black jackets, white shirts and black ties, and in walked Eric. Full lemon-coloured suit, open shirt and a pair of box-fresh Nike sneakers. 'Bloody hell,' we all said. 'The boss is going to kill him.' Alex walked over. Here we go . . . here it comes. 'You look fantastic, Eric.' That was that. But that was Ferguson's genius.

He managed the individual. He got players. Yes, football is a team game, but the boss had this gift for working with the different characters within it. That was the big difference between Alex and Kevin. Kevin was a great motivator of football teams, but Alex could work with individuals. He wanted to understand each part of his team. I knew very quickly that I now had a manager who wanted to know what made me tick.

I'm not the easiest of guys to get on with, quiet, introspective, but my silence at Newcastle was too often misinterpreted, and I think it even intimidated Kevin. Not Alex, he was bang on when it came to managing me. I think people should be comfortable around someone's quietness, and I needed a manager who was interested enough in what was behind that silence. That's what I got. Suddenly I was working with a man I could truly communicate with.

The manager, his staff, my team-mates, the fans – they

were all brilliant. The supporters were desperate for me to be a success, but I was well aware that my game was going to be scrutinised even more now, and that some people within the game wanted to see me fail.

United were in a title race and Blackburn Rovers weren't going to go away. They had spent plenty of money. The £5 million they'd paid for Chris Sutton didn't seem to be a big deal compared to my move. I'd have to get used to being under the microscope. This was Manchester United and so I'd have to get used to it quickly.

Goals came fairly readily, including one in the Manchester derby and a five-goal haul at home to Ipswich when everything went in, but what was happening for the first time was that I was thinking, and thinking isn't always the best thing a striker can do. I don't know if it was Kiddo's words, the change of style or the scrutiny I was under, but I was no longer playing off the cuff.

We had lost at Anfield in March and were second, but we always felt we would catch Blackburn, that the pressure would get to them. I scored important goals at Leicester and Coventry and also in the penultimate game at home to Southampton on the Wednesday, which we won 2–1. So it came to the last game of the season. We would travel to West Ham; Blackburn had to go to Liverpool. We needed to win, with Blackburn getting no better than a draw. It was the longest week of my life.

*

Shirley was about to have a baby, so I had been in London before the Southampton game, but the baby hadn't come. The boss called me and while he never made any demands on me, I felt under pressure. The Premier League was at stake, the title I'd been bought to help win. This, though, was my first child. Could I miss the birth?

My mind scrambled, I caught the shuttle back to Manchester, went home, showered, changed, got to Old Trafford, heard that I had a son (I'd missed his birth!), played the game, scored and went straight back to London. It was a whirlwind. Looking back, it was a mistake, I should have missed that game, but at the time the pressure I felt to win the title was so intense, I made the wrong decision.

Not that I was distracted in the deciding match itself. The game at West Ham was one we thought we could win and we had no time for the talk going around that Liverpool would somehow not play at their best. West Ham went ahead, but we got an equaliser through Brian McClair and then laid siege to their goal. News trickled through that Liverpool were holding Blackburn, but you don't focus on that. I was getting chances, but the keeper, Ludek Miklosko, was making saves. Stuff that.

Give me the ball again. I wasn't going to hide. I have never hidden. Another chance. Give me another chance.

You never think the keeper has got the upper hand, that it's his day, but it became ridiculous. Chance after chance, and this man was making himself huge, saving everything. He was possessed. Nothing was getting past him. He could never play that well again, but that was that. Blackburn had lost at Liverpool, but we couldn't – I couldn't – get the winning goal. The whole season's work, gone in an afternoon.

The tight dressing room at Upton Park was sombre. The manager was upset, but not with us, he couldn't fault our effort. Paul Ince was the most vocal. '**** it,' he said, pacing the room. 'We come back next season and we win it by twenty points!' Next season at United wouldn't come for Incey, but that was something for the future. I needed a holiday.

In London, I held my son and looked into his eyes. 'If you knew what your dad had been through in the last ten days . . .' I whispered. I was drained. I was devastated. I took it all on myself. I had let everyone down. I blamed myself for the title not returning to Old Trafford. I had let down my missus; she was upset. I had let down my son by not being at his birth. I felt everyone's disappointment.

7

TOYS FOR MY BOY

It ended up in a box of toys. A shiny trinket among my one-year-old son Devante's cuddly playthings; among the cars, the trains and the musical instruments. There it sat. My first Premier League winner's medal. My first medal. Devante loved it. Maybe he liked how it shone in the light, who knows, but I was more than happy for him to have it.

One year earlier, when Devante was born, the same week that Blackburn beat Manchester United to the Premier League title, life wasn't easy. The weeks that followed the end of the season were no easier and I went into the new campaign an unsettled man.

But, through hard work (both physical and mental), I managed to settle into that massive club, and together we would take the title from Blackburn's trophy cabinet and from under the noses of my old lot at Newcastle. It had been a mad twelve months, and now, my baby son had a new toy.

*

119

I'd taken a lot of stick for the West Ham result and I was so disappointed about losing the title. On top of that, my personal life wasn't ideal. Shirley and I were new parents and all should have been good, but the fact that I had missed Devante's birth was making things hard and she was in no mood to let it slide. She was seriously upset: 'I'll never forgive you.' Her words hung over me like a cloud.

When you see someone you care about so upset, it hurts and you think of the damage you've done. I'd chosen football over my child. It wasn't like that, but that's how she felt then, and my guilt was affecting me every day. I attempted to explain that I was only trying to work hard so that my family could prosper and that it was simply a gamble that backfired.

Neither the gaffer nor the club had pressurised me to play that night against Southampton. I thought I could do both. I had been signed to help get United over the line, to win the title. I was young and didn't want to let people down. I was trying to do the best for my club and for my family. It had gone wrong, but I was damned if I did and damned if I didn't. I took the decision to play and in the end it went wrong. On both counts. We lost the title and I missed Devante's birth. That summer it weighed on my mind.

My mind had been scrambled for a bit. I've mentioned that towards the end of the 1994–95 season I had been thinking too much. I am a deep thinker anyway, but when it came to football, I had a release. Whatever was going on in my life or my head away from the game, as soon as I got my boots on, I could forget about it. Out on the pitch, apart from central defenders, I didn't have a care in the world.

But things had changed. Even on the pitch I was thinking about things. I was thinking about my football too, thinking about taking chances. I needed to get back to instinct. I am my own worst critic and always will be, but my constant inner doubts, on top of what was being said about the title race and the game at West Ham, was eroding my self-belief. Something had to change.

It was my team-mate Lee Sharpe who noticed I might not be happy, and he told me about a lady he knew who might be able to help. I guess you could call her a guru. Her name was Claire Howell and she ran a course on 'The Secret of Positive Thinking'. It was just what I needed. I saw her for nigh on six months and we worked on getting back my natural confidence. She had me write out affirmations, where I wanted to get to; how to self-motivate, self-believe and get back to the confident footballer I had always been before.

She would come to my house, we would talk, she would show me videos of people sharing their experiences. Nothing to do with football. Lawyers, doctors, business people, all talking about what they go through, how they had lost confidence and how they got it back. It was humbling but empowering and ultimately very helpful. It was step by step, but eventually I got back to where I needed to be.

The fact that Sharpy and I had even had that conversation is mad, because back then, in football, players didn't really talk about that stuff, and any treatment deemed new or different was frowned upon. Football is a man's game and you have to do this and do that, and feel this and feel that.

No one else at the club knew about it. It was my business. I didn't even go to the gaffer. Fergie was brilliant, he was great at moving with the times, and he was the best at managing individuals, but back then, things like talking to an outsider, a guru, well, it wasn't on and so I kept it to myself.

Mental health is very much a talking point in the game today and I'm 100 per cent behind that. Players today get the same sort of stick that we did. It's a game. You win some, you lose some, but then some pen-pusher (or these days keyboard warrior) is telling you where you went wrong, most of them having never played the game. There are plenty of writers you respect, who clearly know the game, but with some, it can be hard to take and it can get to you.

One thing I didn't have to contend with was social

Butter wouldn't melt! Don't be fooled, though. I was often getting into trouble at school.

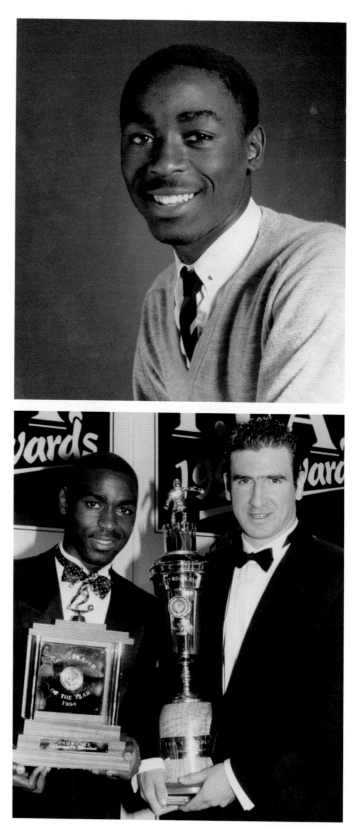

A proud moment: winning the 1993–94 Young Player of the Year award and basking in the glory with future team-mate Eric Cantona, who had won the main award.

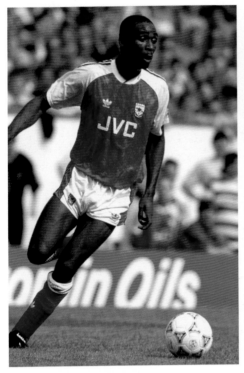

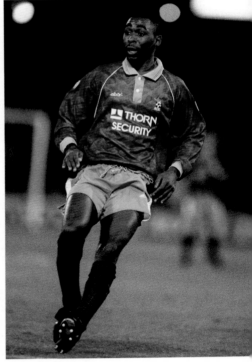

Gunner Cole . . . but my opportunities at Arsenal were limited.

I love Bristol City! It was there that I came alive as a professional footballer in 1992.

Wrong-footing United's Bryan Robson during my Newcastle days.

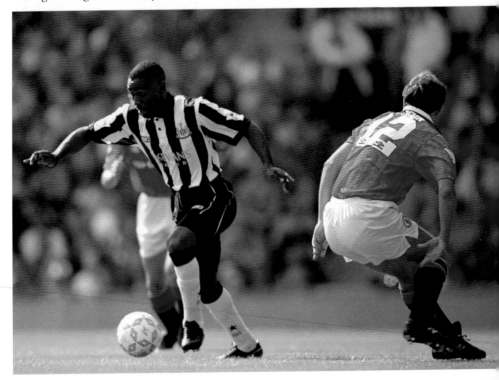

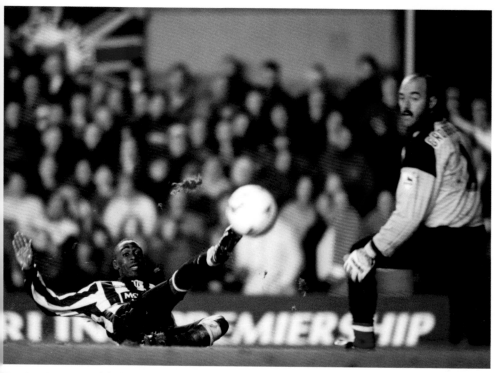

Beating Bruce Grobbelaar for one of three goals against Liverpool in November 1993.

Alex Ferguson welcomes me to Manchester United in 1995 after a transfer I never sought.

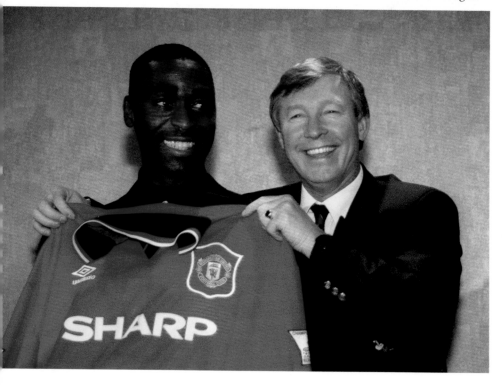

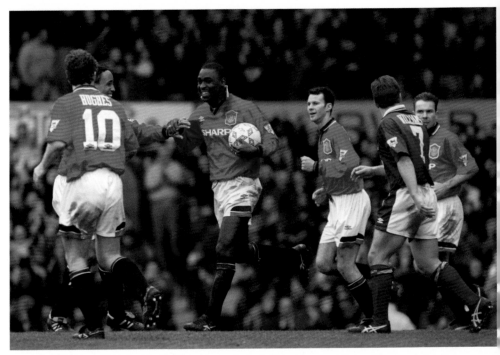

Smiles all round after one of my five goals in United's 9–0 mauling of Ipswich in 1995.

Gary Pallister and Roy Keane in hot pursuit after my goal at Middlesbrough helps wrap up the 1995–96 Premier League title.

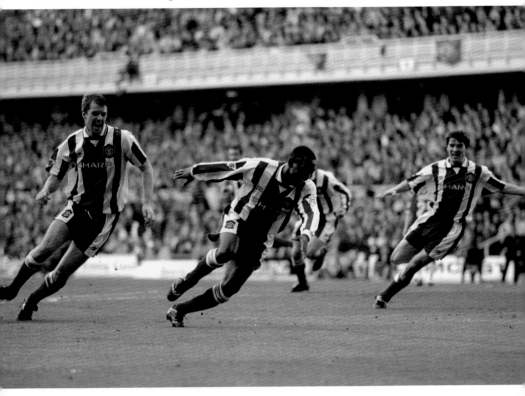

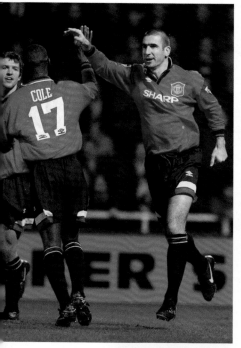

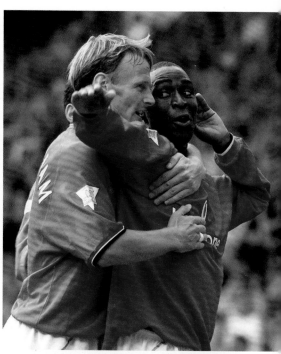

Above left: Eric Cantona, catalyst for so many of United's successes under Sir Alex.

Above right: Teddy Sheringham hugs me after a goal for United, but we never did kiss and make up.

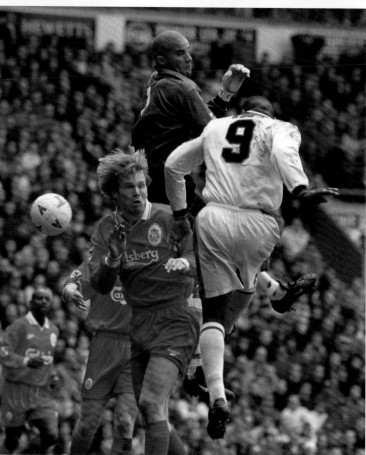

Right: My header finishes off Liverpool at Anfield en route to the 1996–97 Premier League title.

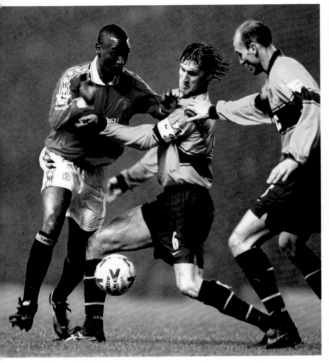

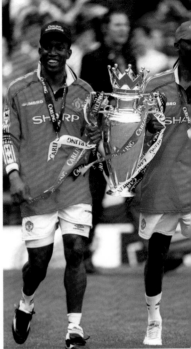

Tussling with Arsenal's Tony Adams and Steve Bould in 1998–99, United's Treble season.

The Treble, part one: revelling in United's Premier League title succes with Dwight and his constant smile

I've just scored against Spurs to seal the first leg of the Treble, and Dwight Yorke and Ryan Giggs want to celebrate!

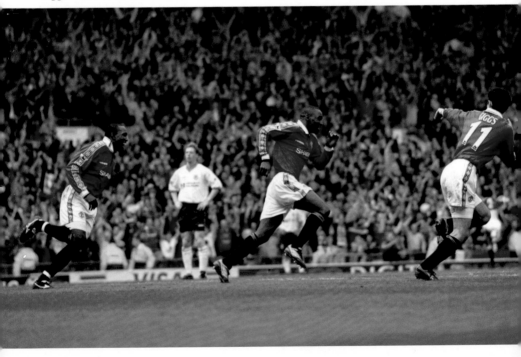

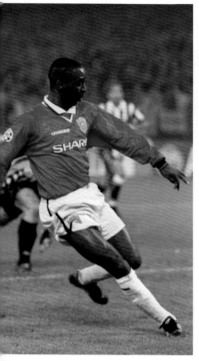

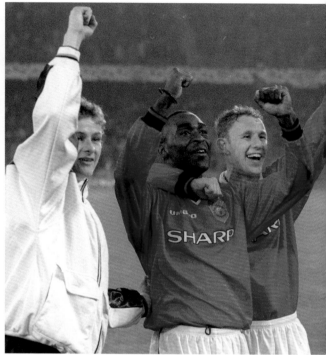

My late goal completes the fightback against Juventus in Turin and we're Barcelona-bound.

Ole Gunnar Solskjaer, myself and Nicky Butt hail our fantastic fans in Turin after our semi-final win.

The Treble, part two: savouring United's FA Cup success with the gaffer and Dwight.

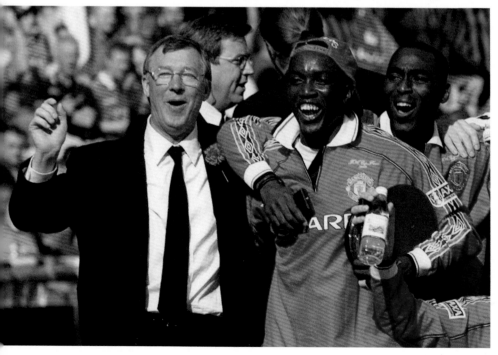

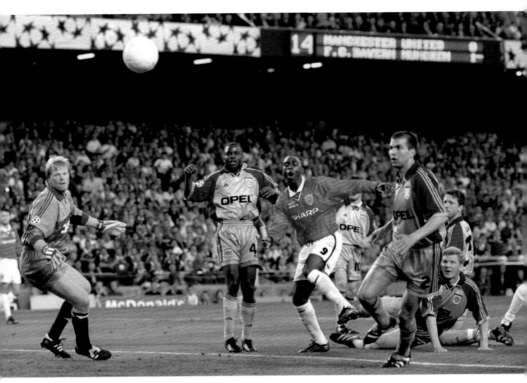

So close against Bayern in Barcelona, before Ole replaced me . . . and scored the winner.

The Treble, part three: we've won the Champions League and it's time to sing our hearts out.

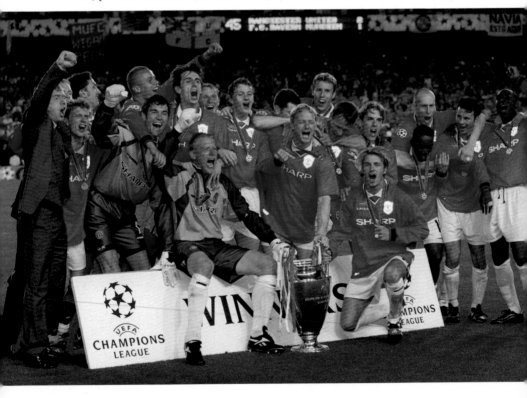

media. Thank God. It can be hard, even at the top of the game where the riches are massive, but I love that players today can feel comfortable talking about their issues, because I don't care who you are, you will have them. Young players, middle-aged players or players coming to the end of their careers, you're going to feel it.

I know a very high-profile player who recently said to me – after I had spoken publicly about my depression following my kidney transplant – that he had everything, medals, money, the lifestyle, the wife, the kids, but sometimes he just sits alone at home and feels only emptiness. 'What the fuck is it all about?' he asked.

As I have said, football was my release, but it was a time when what some would call *real life* was causing me to over-think things. I was living with my agent while I had a new house built. Shirley and Devante would come and stay and ultimately move up to our new home in Wilmslow, in Cheshire, and to be honest, I found my new set-up hard to adjust to.

Shirley's mum moved back to Jamaica. My parents weren't close to Shirley. My dad wasn't having her, despite her Jamaican background. They just didn't get on, so there was another fire I felt I had to put out.

Any new parent will tell you that there is a lot to adjust to and I was no different. I was a hands-on dad, Devante came everywhere with me, and I adored him.

It was a new set-up, though. I was used to living alone, and I know I can be hard to live with. I like things in their place and I had to change because I had a family now. I know Shirley must have found it hard too, because I can drift into my own world, not saying much, just thinking. That caused problems, more fires to put out. It would settle down, but at the time it was difficult, and I also had a new football season to think of.

I had an operation that summer to sort out shin splints, and was eager to right the previous season's wrongs, but it would be with a slightly new team. When I had signed in the January, there had been no talk of the gaffer rebuilding his great side, but come the start of the campaign, Mark Hughes had gone, Paul Ince had gone and Andrei Kanchelskis was seeking a move away.

Sparky and Ince were big characters, big personalities, and would be missed. I thought Sparky would sign a new short-term deal, but he went and Incey was off to Italy. He'd been great with me when I arrived, regularly having me over for dinner with his family.

I'm not that interested in Incey's persona. All that Guv'nor stuff wasn't the real him, and he actually wanted to distance himself from it. All the bravado, the outgoing stuff, I don't judge people on all that. Sit down and have a one-on-one conversation with me and then I'll make up my mind. Incey was brilliant with me and, as a very good player, I thought he was going to be a big loss.

I had seen first-hand this new crop of young players coming through the ranks, a group that would be called 'the Class of '92', including the Neville brothers, Paul Scholes, David Beckham, Nicky Butt and Ryan Giggs. On top of their talent, you could see that their work rate and attitude was spot on. They had the club's ethos ingrained in them. They all knew what it took to make it at Manchester United and they had this scary drive to succeed. But you don't know how good a young player will really be until they get a run in the team.

With Sparky gone, and Eric suspended, Scholesy would come in and play up front. He was some forward as a kid, able to play as a centre-forward or in the hole off me. He had that football IQ I talked about with Peter Beardsley. I'd be lying if I said that I thought at the time he'd become one of the best midfielders the club had ever seen, but that's what happened.

The Neville brothers were very good. The talk then was that Phil was the better player, but with Gary, I have never seen a footballer work harder to improve or to get to where he did. Talent alone isn't enough, and through sheer graft, Gary had the better career.

Talking of hard work, David Beckham. Who knew

back then that he would become this global phenom-
enon, but as with Gary, the work he put into his
football was crazy. After training he'd be out on his
own, crossing, crossing, crossing (he became the best
crosser of the ball I've ever seen). Free-kicks for hours.
That was how those guys got to the very top.

Then there was Butty, a tenacious, brilliant midfielder,
great engine. He'd put his foot in, but he could play as
well. Others who didn't make it, like Ben Thornley and
Chris Casper, were good players too, but unlucky with
injuries. It was an exciting crop of footballers.

I was only a few years older than them, don't forget.
My career path was very different from theirs but we
were all desperate to do well at the club, and I got on
well with them all. I'd go with Giggsy for nights out
and we always had a laugh. The strength and the ultimate success of this new Manchester United squad lay
in how well the youngsters integrated with the senior
players, and I think the gaffer could see from the way
these lads, during the previous season, had contributed
to the team and the dressing room that now was the
right time to make them regulars.

One game into the new season, though, and plenty
might have thought he was wrong. We were beaten
comprehensively by a good, experienced Aston Villa

team. I didn't play, as I hadn't yet got clearance from the surgeon who carried out my operation, but the 3–1 scoreline was clearly a fair result and the whole squad took it on the chin. No panic.

It was the media who were all over it and, of course, it was Alan Hansen, the BBC pundit, who made his famous comment that in football you can't win anything with kids. Alan has been battered for those words, but I think what he meant was that, because of the big players and big personalities we had lost, the gaffer needed to spend a few quid on seasoned pros.

What he couldn't see behind the scenes was the way the squad had gelled, how well the young players had come in and settled, and how well the senior pros had both accepted and helped them. When you have a squad with the likes of Peter Schmeichel, Brucie, Pally, Denis Irwin, Roy Keane and Eric, you are talking about mad experience and mad leadership qualities.

That team could have had any number of captains, but what we all knew, the kids included, was that once you crossed that white line, you were your own skipper. Navigate your own ship. Yes, you're working with a team, but get your game right, meet the standards asked of you, and the team will be OK.

The dressing room was unbelievable. No one was scared to pipe up or say their bit. The youngsters too. Roy Keane was never shy, even as a younger man. That's what I liked about him. That's what I liked about the dressing room. Some were louder than others, but there wasn't one shrinking violet. If there were arguments, and there were arguments, it would be sorted in the right way without anyone thinking their opinion didn't count.

After Villa, we won our next five games. Scholes was scoring. Sharpy, Giggsy, Becks, all of us were showing how good this team might become. But there had been something missing. Eric Cantona. It was what it was: he couldn't play and we had to get on with things. We had really missed him the previous season, but with Scholesy doing so well, it had been OK so far this season, but once the ban was over, it was clear he was going to come straight back in.

The media circus around him was nuts. Front-page journalists were now as interested in him as the sports guys. We got on with things but the harassment was so bad, I think Eric and the gaffer wondered if it would be better if he left. Inter Milan were very keen, but how could United lose him? This genius. This mercurial talent who just seemed the perfect fit for the English game.

In France, they weren't having him. He'd upset too many people, and who knows if the Italian game would have suited his one-off style? There was something about him and the English game. The English fans loved having him here. The collars up, the mad goals, the swagger.

He was an enigma. Even attacking the abusive fan, and then the remarks about sardines and trawlers, there was something very different about Eric and this country fell for him.

And what a footballer. Big, a strong man, barrel-chested, great on the ball, able to do the unexpected. I hadn't had the chance to play much football with him, but now he was back and the whole country was watching.

To add to the razzmatazz, Eric's first game back was against Liverpool at Old Trafford. It was a hard game. Liverpool were improving and Robbie Fowler, a great young player, got two goals to put them 2–1 up. It was always going to be Eric's day, though, and he equalised from the spot, before swinging on the goal stanchion in celebration. Typical Eric.

I've mentioned just how good the gaffer was with Eric, how brilliantly he managed the individual, and they didn't come much more individual than Eric. With this new squad, I got to see just how much of a genius Fergie was. He had twenty-one players, different ages, different characters, different egos, different families, with different problems, but he was on top of all of it. Whatever was happening, he was there, helping, guiding, giving out bollockings. Genius.

And he knew everything. One night I'd been out, nothing wild, but I was driving home late and I passed an overturned car. I went straight to the nearest police station to report it. A day or two later, the gaffer asked me, 'What were you doing out so late the other night?' How did he know?

It turns out it was his friend who had had the accident. He gave me a bit of a hard time but then he said, 'Well done.' I'd done the right thing. He could be your counsellor, your boss, your friend, a father figure, and once with me he was a lawyer too.

Before a game at Old Trafford, he'd come to me and said, 'We need to talk after the game, son.'

No we don't, I was nervously thinking.

After the match, he pulled me to one side. Here we go.

'Son, you need to talk to the Flying Squad.'

Now, I hadn't done anything and I was thinking, what is going on?

'No, I don't.'

'Yes, you do.'

It turns out an old mate of mine who used to come and see the games had got himself into a bit of bother and the police wanted to question me. I wasn't in trouble myself, but it might still have been a nasty experience. The gaffer said he'd come with me for the interview and he sat in the room with the Old Bill, calming everything down, putting me at ease and making sure it all went smoothly. It was unbelievable what he did to protect his players.

That meant he never, ever dug us out in public. When talking to the press after a game, if I was criticised he would go on the attack, turning it around, saying, 'Are you sure? The lad should have won us two penalties.' Or it was the ref. Then, a few minutes later, he'd be in the dressing room tearing absolute strips off me, letting me know how bad I'd been.

Fergie used to say to us that if any of us ever went into management, we should follow his lead and never criticise our players in public. However frustrated, however bad they'd been, never go after them to the press, because you're going to need them the following Saturday.

The dressing room was a fiery place. I wasn't afraid to give it back to the gaffer and we would have some right good rows. I think he respected how much I'd back myself, but he also got me, got my methods, how I liked to train. 'You could start a fight in an empty house,' he'd say with a smile, and he was right. The gaffer understood me and he would work with each of us individually. He was the most amazing manager. Fergie never met my dad – that would have been interesting – but he had a similar influence on my life and you never stop learning from someone like that.

*

I was learning all the time. At Newcastle, I'd been the main man, and I was used to one way of playing. Make my runs, explode into space behind defenders and get in that way. Now I was being asked to be an all-round striker. Early on at Manchester United, I'd make a little run in and the ball wouldn't come. That was a half-decent run, I'd be thinking, but the team wasn't programmed that way. I had to link play, play with my back to goal, yes, get on the end of things, but also add to my game. Brian Kidd worked and worked with me as I tried to become a better footballer.

In the meantime, my old mates at Newcastle had moved on and with Les Ferdinand doing great things in my place, they were the front runners in the Premier League and, with a big lead at Christmas, looked like the favourites.

Clarky would be on the phone to me, giving it good banter like he always does, and with Newcastle having an eleven-point lead at one point, I couldn't really be giving it back. We were beaten 4–1 at Tottenham on New Year's Day, but from there we went on the sort of run the gaffer relished. There was loads of talk about Newcastle's leaky defence, but he was only ever fussed about us and with that focus our results put us right on Kevin Keegan's radar.

The gaffer had knowledge. 'The season doesn't start until Easter,' he'd say. That made me laugh, but what he meant was that you get your hard work done, and then with the fixtures piling up alongside the pressure, points would be dropped and any lead chased down.

The gaffer had experience. Even I, a newcomer, had been part of the title run the year before, while other than Peter Beardsley, no player at Newcastle knew what it was like to try to get over the line.

The gaffer also had Eric. On our winning run, Eric was on fire. We would win games 1–0, with Eric constantly getting the decisive goal, and in March it was Eric who scored the goal that won the game at Newcastle, a win that blew the title race wide open.

It was a massive night. My first match back at St James', and there was animosity towards me. Nothing I couldn't handle, and you half expect it. Anyway, I had a job to do for Manchester United and we all went into the game knowing we could win. Knowing we had to win.

Eric got the goal but the night belonged to Schmeichel. He was brilliant. With save after save, he thwarted the Newcastle efforts. He was worth a good sixteen points a season on his own and that night we might have lost 4–1 without him.

Peter was some character. Loud. Demanding. Always wanting more from us and even more from himself. You could hear him at the training ground before you saw him. He'd constantly be on us at training, and in games. At first I found him a bit much. All that noise. Not for me. As I got to know the man, though, I liked him. He was cool, and the important thing to know is no goalkeeper is the full ticket anyway.

Out of everyone, Peter was probably the easiest to wind up. He was meticulous about his towels and his gloves. He'd have six towels in a pile and his gloves all lined up. Do not touch his towels and, whatever you do, do not go near his gloves. Of course, we did and that's when the big man would go nuts.

'Where are my gloves?' he'd shout. I can hear him now. That big booming voice.

'WHERE ARE MY ******* GLOVES?'

Peter symbolised the whole dressing room. Defeat wasn't accepted. That's why we scored so many late goals, and with that belief, we continued to push for the title and put pressure on Keegan and his team, before eventually overtaking them.

I scored in a big win at Manchester City and we won tight games, thanks as ever to Eric, at home to Arsenal and then Spurs. Even when we did lose, the manager found a way of deflecting the setback. We'd played rubbish at Southampton. We were 3–0 down at half-time and walked into the dressing room ready to have the riot act read to us. The gaffer sat us down.

'Right, get that **** kit off,' he said.

We'd been playing in our grey away strip and Fergie

wanted us in the blue one instead. None of us liked the grey kit and Fergie thought it was hard for us to pick each other out. That wasn't true. We were just playing badly, but there it was. We won the second half 1–0 and the gaffer had his excuse to give the press. Once again, genius.

We didn't dwell on that loss, beating Leeds at home, where Keane scored a big winner, before a 5–0 win at home to Nottingham Forest put us on the verge of taking the title. Newcastle had struggled to live with the pressure. That inexperience was telling. Fergie had made a few remarks in the press, questioning whether teams would try as hard against Newcastle as they did against us, and it was soon clear the gaffer had got inside Kevin's head.

Kevin's rant became infamous. His 'I will love it if we beat them' speech played again and again, but at the time it was clear to us that we'd won the title. I knew Kevin well. I've mentioned how emotional he could be as a manager, but this was a time for calm. Kevin's heart was on his sleeve. It's what made him so effective at times, but on this occasion his emotions let him down. Throwing a wobbly transmits to your players.

In contrast, we had a manager who loved chasing teams down, who knew a thing or two about pacing his teams just right. I watched Kevin on telly that night, and while I always respected him, I didn't have any sympathy. You can't. I was a Manchester United player. On the other side of the coin. Newcastle were the opposition. They were trying to win something that I was desperate to win, and seeing Kevin lose it meant we were likely to do just that.

Our last game was at Middlesbrough. I scored in a 3–0 win and the Premier League was won. What a difference a year makes. After the disappointment at West Ham and the troubles I'd had getting my mind right, I was a champion of England.

That's what matters. Moments like that define a team. Define a career. You can have all the money in the world, but once you're playing at the highest level, it's the medals and the trophies you have won that count. If you end your career without winning anything, that is a massive disappointment. I'd worked so hard to be here, gone through ups and big downs, but now I had that medal.

Not that the season was over. As ever, we'd gone on a good FA Cup run. I'd scored a last-minute winner at Sunderland in the third round, and got the equaliser against Chelsea in the semi at Villa Park. Becks got the winner that day and so we were off to Wembley for the chance to win the Double.

We were up against Liverpool. They had given us big

problems in both the league games, beating us 2–0 at Anfield. Fowler was having a mad season and in Steve McManaman they had a brilliant forward with a free role to roam about the pitch. I think it was him who worried the gaffer, who wanted Keane to play a deeper role in front of our back four to keep him quiet.

What wasn't quiet was Liverpool's pre-match attire. The cream suits raised a lot of eyebrows and when it came to giving his team talk, Fergie was straight on it. 'Look at those suits they're wearing,' he said. 'They think they've won this.' I think their keeper, David James, had done some modelling with Armani and sorted out the suits, but they weren't good.

If you wear something like that, you'd better play the game of your life, but the truth is neither side could say they did that. It was a terrible game. One of the worst I was ever involved in. Maybe it was the intense rivalry, but both teams seemed terrified of defeat.

It was Eric once again who settled things with a late goal after a mistake from James, and so we had the FA Cup to go with the Premier League. We'd won the Double. We took a lap of honour in front of our amazing fans, fans who had backed me all the way and who now cheered this new, exciting team from the pitch. It had been a crazy five years since I had left Arsenal, but now I had everything I wanted from the game. And my son had his new toys.

8
NO CHANCE!

A washout. That's how I'd describe my international career. If I was to explain it to my dad, a cricket fan, I'd liken myself to a batsman, fully padded up, sitting in the pavilion waiting for the clouds to lift and the umpires to give me the nod. Unfortunately, when it came to England and me, the covers never really came off.

Fifteen caps and one goal is nowhere near a total to match my dreams and ambitions, and it says a lot about the stuttering, stop-start nature of my time with England that my first four caps were given to me over four years by four different managers.

When I was growing up I was adamant that I would be a professional footballer. I played the game because I loved it, and that passion meant I could never see myself doing anything else. Teachers would ask what I wanted to be, and would politely smile when I said a footballer. Some might have thought prison was a more likely path for me, but I knew that I would get there.

With all that hope and drive to do well, of course you think of playing for your country. You want to make it into the club game and then, if you're good enough, you think of getting your international chance. Those thoughts never changed, but with time and experience I realised that, however well I played at club level, getting a chance with England, and I mean a real good crack at it, was asking way too much, and when I look back on it now, it feels very incomplete.

It looked like it would be so different. I was a poster boy for the FA. I played and scored goals at every single level. I was selected for Lilleshall, schoolboy international, under-16s, under-17s, under-21s. I was enthusiastic and ambitious. I understood that I had to give my best for my club and, with that hard work, England was a more than welcome bonus.

I can hear my under-21 manager Lawrie McMenemy's big Geordie voice telling us all, 'Just work hard, and do what you do with your clubs.' It was a simple message. I loved the under-21s. No politics, no lies, just ambitious young players being rewarded for their hard work with international football.

We used to love big Lawrie. He took some stick off us all, though. We were young and a bit mean. He used to waddle about the place and we'd joke about his huge head. Always behind his back, of course. We had too much respect for him to say anything to him. He was scary, too, and anyway, if you did get caught, you knew you were going home. They were legendary days. I liked Lawrie a lot.

One day, in 1993, he came to my room, stood in the doorway and said, 'Pack your bags, son.'

He had his stern look on his face and I was standing there thinking, 'What have I done?' I was racking my brain to think of what I might have said and who might have grassed on me.

Lawrie let me suffer for a bit before breaking into a big smile and saying, 'Congratulations, you've been called up into the senior squad.'

I couldn't believe it. A year earlier I had been playing for Bristol City at Grimsby Town in front of 5,000 fans but, thanks to my move to Newcastle and the goals I had immediately started to score in the Premier League, I was an England player. I was buzzing.

The senior squad itself was less upbeat. Under Graham Taylor, qualification for the 1994 World Cup had stalled. England lost in Holland on a mad night when the officials did so much to frustrate the team. 'Do I not like that?' became a national catchphrase and you couldn't blame Taylor for his remarks after the Dutch defender Ronald Koeman should have been sent off for a foul on David Platt and then, minutes later, curled one in the top bin to effectively end any hopes of going to America for the tournament.

The knives were out for the manager and the players, but when I arrived I was in awe, apprehensive about what to expect. I went straight to my room and I didn't come out. Not until there was a knock on the door. It was Des Walker and Carlton Palmer. 'Come on, you're coming out with us,' they said, and I'll always be grateful for how much they helped me settle in, taking me out for a few drinks with the lads and making me feel like I belonged.

It was another example of how much senior pros can help younger players. I had it at Arsenal, at Bristol City, Newcastle and Manchester United, and that night with England. I immediately enjoyed being around these guys, listening to them, getting a feel for what it's like to be a full international.

I was an unused sub for the last group game, a 7–1 win against San Marino, but my appetite for more had got bigger. What was clear was that any future with England I had would be with a new manager. I felt for Graham Taylor. He was a good footballing man, passionate, he was straight up and he didn't deserve anywhere near the sort of stick he took from what had become a gutter press.

You could see the sort of pressure Graham was under, and the savage treatment in some of the papers opened my eyes to just how low parts of the press would go. A man tries to do his job to the best of his ability. Sometimes it doesn't go right, but that is by no means an excuse to decimate him as a man. That's not on and to see him almost dehumanised was hard. I think I certainly started to mistrust the press then.

England had failed to reach a World Cup and that tarnished everyone involved. For me, an outsider getting his first taste of it all, I had my own frustrations. I had scored plenty of goals prior to those England games, and Graham had said to me that, should they qualify, I had every chance of going to the World Cup.

I went on to score those forty-one goals that season, and without being big-headed, there is no way I could have been left out, not after that season. It's a massive case of *what if*. I had always dreamt of playing in a World Cup, but instead I watched the tournament on the telly, hoping that my time would soon come.

Euro '96 was the next tournament on the horizon and the new manager was Terry Venables. I didn't know Terry at all. He was a stranger to me and as he announced his first few squads without me in them, it seemed that's what he would remain.

I was still scoring goals for Newcastle, not as many as the season before, but repeating that level of success was never going to happen. I thought I deserved a chance. The manager thought otherwise. Then one day Kevin asked me into his office at the training ground. David Davies, the FA's head of communications, was on the phone. Kevin had his feet up on the desk as he beckoned me in to listen to David talk about how Terry thought I was struggling with my fitness, that I looked sluggish and wasn't right for the squad right now.

I was shocked. Right there in that room, at that moment, I realised that my international career was going to be an uphill run. Terry had said in the press that despite England only playing friendlies for a couple of years, because of qualifying as hosts, he wasn't going to hand out caps like confetti. It was a line that stuck with me.

At the start of the 1994–95 season my Newcastle team-mates Peter Beardsley and Barry Venison got called up – and rightly so, they were both playing brilliantly – but I was overlooked again and again. It wasn't until I had moved to Manchester United that I was finally selected. England were playing Uruguay in March 1995 and I started that month scoring five goals against Ipswich. Not even Terry could talk about me being sluggish after that.

It should have been the best night of my footballing life. I was on the bench, but when Terry gave me the nod, I rushed to get my tracksuit off, excited that I might break the deadlock in a tight 0–0 match, and that I was about to win the full cap I had always wanted. This is it.

Instead it was a damp squib, and the start of a feud with a team-mate that would go on for years. Teddy Sheringham was a player I looked up to. A senior player with plenty of caps, goals and experience. For all the respect I had for him, he was far from pleased to see his number come up and instead of greeting me on the sideline to wish me luck or congratulate me, he dejectedly walked off, twenty-five yards down the touchline, without even looking at me, let alone acknowledging my moment.

I was astounded. I couldn't get my head around his attitude or the selfishness of his act. I ran onto the pitch and instead of feeling pride, I felt embarrassed, belittled – as if what I was about to achieve, what I had always dreamt of achieving, actually meant nothing.

That might sound like an overreaction to some. Why should I let another player's actions affect my big moment? But when you have dreamt of something for so long, when you have pictured it, and part of that picture is the respect from your team-mates for doing it, to have all that taken ruined it for me, and I could not forgive Teddy for what he did that night.

As I grew older, I always tried to be a good pro. I tried to look out for younger players and give them advice, think about what they were going through. This was partly because I had the pleasure of being looked out for by great pros like David O'Leary, Paul Davis, Leroy Rosenior and Peter Beardsley, but it was also partly because of Teddy's actions at Wembley.

The match itself was a nothing. I hated every minute of it. I couldn't get the negativity of my start out of my head. I actually hit the bar, but all I can remember is wanting to get off the pitch. Was this what it was all about? I didn't expect a big fuss, but it felt like Teddy had looked down on me and I left the squad with nothing but a bad taste in my mouth. More disappointments would follow with England, but that first one always stayed with me.

I wasn't surprised to be left out of Terry's squad for the 1996 Euros. It was clear he didn't fancy me. Winning the Double with Manchester United that year wasn't going to change that, and at no point, despite making my debut, did I have any hopes that I would be picked.

I watched it, of course. Mates were playing in it and, like the whole country, I was excited about how well the team were playing. People might expect a player who hasn't made the squad to spend the summer jealously avoiding the football, but I was fine. When it's simply a case of the manager not rating you, it's easier to take.

If I had played loads for Terry and then been dropped

at the last minute then, yes, that would have been hard to take, but ever since listening to that message from David Davies while at Newcastle, I sensed I wasn't one for Terry and just told myself to focus on Manchester United and take it from there. It had been announced that Terry would be leaving after the tournament, so I had to look forward to a clean slate that I could make my mark on.

Glenn Hoddle was next, and like Terry I didn't know him other than having watched him as a kid and always respected him as a player. I didn't have any major conversations with Glenn, but I got into a few squads, kept my head down, worked hard for my club and waited for a chance.

In the summer of 1997 I was picked for the squad for the Tournoi competition in France and really enjoyed being around a tournament situation. My game time was minimal, though, and when that happens you do start to doubt whether this manager fancies you and wonder why you're there.

Glenn wasn't the best communicator. He wasn't particularly good at transmitting his messages to the players. He could show you, he liked to show you, but if you didn't live up to his high standards, it was a case of 'Oh what, you can't do that?'

He just expected you to be this or that, but that's not enough. I won't apologise for using Sir Alex Ferguson as an example of how to manage, because he was the best I worked with, and the gaffer was brilliant at making you feel you could do anything. He really could communicate and with his words in your ear, you'd feel a million dollars. That's man-management. Glenn lacked those skills.

I learnt that the hard way when, before the 1998 World Cup, he publicly slated me, saying, 'Cole needs four or five chances before he scores.' It was an unfortunate comment and it hurt. I was playing for Manchester United, I was scoring goals, winning Premier Leagues, playing against the best defenders in world football, making a ripple in Europe, so to hear the national team manager telling people I needed too many chances was disrespectful and ultimately ignorant.

And there it was. Another obstacle. Another England manager who had made up his mind about me. My chances of going to the World Cup in France had slipped away. Glenn picked his squad and the strikers going were Alan Shearer, Michael Owen, Teddy Sheringham and Les Ferdinand. Ian Wright and Dion Dublin had made the preliminary squad too. But not me. All of them were brilliant forwards, of course they were, but I felt I had every right to be disappointed.

I had enjoyed a good season with United. Arsenal had won the Double, but on a personal note I was pleased with my overall game. I scored fifteen Premier League goals, I was runner-up to Dennis Bergkamp in the PFA awards and my all-round game had never been better. The United fans had voted me their player of the year, and so talk about how many chances I needed to score a goal was plain stupid.

The teenager Michael Owen had burst onto the scene, Alan Shearer was England's main man, but in terms of form and fitness, I had had a better season than most. Les had only scored five league goals, Teddy had got nine, Wrighty only ten. Alan had missed half the season through injury and only scored twice.

That's what annoyed me about Glenn's comments. Whatever the truth, when an England manager talks, people listen. His words stuck. The official Manchester United magazine ran a piece standing up for me, showing that in the 1997–98 season my fifteen goals came from ninety-one attempts, giving me a success rate of 16.4 per cent. The best ratio from any English striker in the league. There you go, Glenn.

Paul Gascoigne's omission from the squad got all the headlines, but mine came with a short but not sweet phone call from Glenn.

'Hi, Andy,' he said. 'I'm just calling to touch base.'

You could hear it in his voice that it was bad news,

and I wasn't going to hang about and listen to his small talk.

'OK, great, thanks, Glenn. Good luck,' and I put the phone down. That was that.

Impulsive? Maybe, but I wasn't going to listen to it all. Not when he had discredited my whole game in public. He had questioned me as a footballer and there was no way I was going, so why have a nice little chat over the phone? Good luck and see you later.

It was a hard summer. My ambitions were waning. I had had a really good season with my club – everything I had been told to do since coming through the ranks with England – but it wasn't enough. I was learning that there were politics involved. I was learning that managers had their minds set and if your face didn't fit, then you were struggling, big time.

One Sunday morning in the autumn of 1998, it became crystal clear that my mug, while Glenn was in charge, was never going to fit. I drove to a petrol station and picked up a newspaper and was greeted by a back-page headline that read, COLE HEARTBREAK – HE WON'T BE IN THE ENGLAND SQUAD FOR THE NEXT 18 MONTHS. I thought, 'What have I done now?' I opened the paper and was shocked to read Glenn slagging me off again in another interview.

'There has been no significant improvement since the World Cup,' he said. 'He still needs the same amount of chances to score a goal. To see dramatic change would be a year to eighteen months down the line – if it happens.'

I couldn't believe my eyes. I hadn't even gone to the World Cup in which his team failed to get to the quarter-finals, and he's digging *me* out. I'm getting on with my work at my club, I'm not in his plans and that's fine, but don't be going public – for the second time – and making me look stupid. I wasn't having it. Two can play that game.

I did my own interview with *The Sun* to have my say. I called Glenn a coward, asked if he was a man or a mouse. Yes, it was fighting talk, but I wasn't going to be spoken about like that. If he wanted to have an argument in the papers rather than face to face, then fine by me.

The press loved it, of course. Glenn, like any England manager, had his favourites on the papers. The *Mirror*'s Harry Harris had his say, backing Glenn's hypothesis about me. Lee Clayton on the *Daily Star* piped up, saying I couldn't hit a cow's arse with a banjo. That made me laugh. Two weeks later I scored a goal at the Nou Camp that is still talked about today and had Louis van Gaal out of his seat in the Barcelona dug-out. Cow's arses and banjos are one thing, but scoring

Champions League goals in the cathedrals of European football is another.

I was confident in my ability and obviously confident with my arguments, but over two decades later, I can look back and wonder why Glenn had it in for me. He left lots of players out of his squads, but never did he so publicly lay into them, never did he question their actual livelihood. It seemed personal, and that has always confused me, because all I ever did while he was England manager was get my head down and work.

Just weeks later, and ironically because of another interview Glenn gave to the papers, he was sacked and when I heard Kevin Keegan was taking over, my thoughts raced. My face was certainly familiar to the new boss, but there was a history. In football, you hope that there is no baggage; you come across friends and foes and you have to get on with things.

Howard Wilkinson took the team for one friendly – a 2–0 defeat to France at Wembley in February 1999 – but it was Kevin who took the reins, an England legend who immediately had the fans on side. Kevin actually gave me the majority of my fifteen caps and I thank him for that, but once again, it seemed that the chance of a real run of games was going to be hard to come by.

England qualified for the European Championships in Holland and Belgium in 2000, and I had a decision to make. I had had a niggling foot injury and it needed an operation, but this was a major tournament, something I had always wanted to take part in. There was, though, a bigger picture to think about.

My heart and my emotions were screaming to go, but I knew that if I did, and then came back to Old Trafford telling the gaffer I needed an operation prior to the season, I was going to be out for a bit, and if you're out for a bit at Manchester United, you might be out for good.

I dropped out of the squad. Kevin Phillips went to the tournament instead and, even with hindsight, I don't regret it. England didn't have a good time out there, but from my point of view, as a potential squad player, there didn't seem to be much flexibility. The team, the forward line, it didn't change, despite bad results, and I looked on, thinking I would have just sat on the bench. I would have needed to have that operation and then struggled into the following season. Instead, I was raring to go come August and there was now another World Cup to look forward to.

Kevin was giving everything to the England job. As ever, his heart was on his sleeve, but despite his legendary status as an England player, the job isn't easy and results mean everything. Losing at home to Germany when you're already under pressure won't do, and when Liverpool's Didi Hamann scored at Wembley on a damp Saturday afternoon in October 2000, the knives were out.

I started the game up front with Michael Owen, but it was tight, far from inspirational. There weren't many chances and as we walked back to the dressing room in the rain, you could hear the abuse coming Kevin's way. It was hard to watch. Lots had happened between me and Kevin, but I always respected and liked him, and to watch him clearly taking it all in, that was difficult.

Still, I and all the other lads were shocked when he walked into the dressing room and resigned there and then. I've mentioned before how impulsive he could be and how hard he took defeat, but even for him this was a rash decision. Kevin put so much pressure on himself. You could see that, and his desire to succeed in the job was never in doubt. It must have been tough, but he wasn't going to change his mind and, yet again, England were looking for a new manager.

While that search was taking place, Howard Wilkinson took us for a game out in Finland. Howard had been involved prior to Kevin getting the job and I really liked him. He was a cool guy. Knew his stuff. I also liked him because, however briefly he was there, he was the only manager to take me to one side and talk to me. It helped that the words he used were positive.

Before the game in Helsinki he said I was going to start and he talked in a way that made me feel like this was a manager who would have faith in me. By now, Shirley and I had had our second child, a daughter we named Faith, but that wasn't a word I think of much when it comes to my international career, yet the new manager – albeit a caretaker – gave me the shot in the arm I had lacked.

With Howard I felt good, but it was only short-lived. The FA had big plans. Howard wasn't part of them and instead they were going abroad. Sven-Göran Eriksson had an impressive CV, having worked at some of Europe's biggest clubs, and his appointment showed that the FA were now prepared to pay a top salary to get the national team up to the highest level.

Sven was on massive money and the pressure was on to get England to the 2002 World Cup in Japan. I shared that ambition. I was playing well for Manchester United and I was desperate to get to a tournament. I had my doubters, I knew. They had always been there. To them, I simply wasn't good enough for international football. I saw that as rubbish. The fact that I hadn't scored yet for my country was a stick the so-called pundits would beat me with, but plenty of our top strikers had gone long spells without goals and I knew, given that run in the team that I so craved, goals would come.

I was proved right. I started in Sven's first three games, and got my first goal in the last of them, out in Albania in March 2001. I was buzzing. I had scored at every level for England from schoolboy up and now, maybe, I had a manager willing to give me a real chance.

Luck, though, had other ideas. I got booked in Albania, which meant I'd miss the next qualifier. It was a big blow. Looking back, it lost me vital momentum. I played a friendly at the start of the following season, I was on the bench when we famously won 5–1 in Munich in September 2001, I played the second half in the 2–2 draw against Greece at Old Trafford a month later, when Becks had his brilliant moment, and so I was hopeful of getting in the final twenty-two.

In December 2001, I left Manchester United for Blackburn. That wasn't easy, but I was playing well, scoring goals and thought I was in with a chance of making Sven's World Cup squad. I was wrong. In February 2002, England were going to Holland for a friendly, and Sven phoned me.

'Hello, Andy,' he said in his quiet polite way. 'I am going to have a look at a few new faces, but don't worry, you'll be in the next squad.'

I haven't heard from Sven-Göran Eriksson since.

Darius Vassell got in and he went to Japan. Vass was

a great player, and could play on the wing, which he often did, but I'd had enough of it all. This was the World Cup I really believed I'd done more than enough to go to. I'd even been promised a spot in the next squad, had continued to score Premier League goals, but nothing. Not even another call. As far as I was concerned, Sven had been dishonest with me and I found that hard to take.

That's when I decided to pack it in. I'd had enough. It was the last straw and I was angry. What's the point of doing my best, only to be made to sit around and be treated like that? I was fuming and what made things worse was that those same people who had gone on about me not being good enough for international football were now piping up, saying how dare I retire: 'Who does he think he is?'

I'll decide. When it comes to my career, I make the decisions. People can, and do, say exactly what they think about footballers, and you can take that, but don't tell me when I should make the massive decision of retiring from the international game. That was my business and, as I say, enough was enough.

Now that I had retired from international football, I watched England under Sven from a distance and with interest. First of all, the tag 'The Golden Generation' was a nonsense. You have to win something to be called 'Golden' and it is so English to build something up before it succeeds. It's then fun to knock it down. The players didn't ask to have the tag, but it stuck and ultimately they were criticised for it.

'Underachievers' was a term later thrown at them. I don't think that's right either. Yes, they were brilliant players and, yes, they were right to expect to do very well, but what about the teams who beat them? In 2002, even when they lost to Brazil there was a national debate. 'Why have we failed again?' Hold on, they lost to Brazil, the eventual winners, with Ronaldo, Ronaldinho and Rivaldo in their ranks. I've always found that a little disrespectful to the other nations England played.

I could see that England were too often trying to fit square pegs into round holes, and that was never going to work. A manager has to have big enough nuts to leave out good players. That's what you get paid for. The Steven Gerrard and Frank Lampard and Paul Scholes debate has raged on for many years, but it was going to take real strength of character to leave one out when necessary, to play players from the bench, to be flexible with selections, to mix it up, to understand you need subtle change to win tournaments, but too often easy decisions were made and the team suffered.

Players from that time have talked publicly about the pressure of playing for England, the cliques involved and how unenjoyable joining the squad had become. That sounds crazy, but I can vouch for it being true. I didn't feel pressure as such, I was desperate to do well, but the cliques were definitely there and, during the worst times, I actively set out to stay at home.

I'd go to Sir Alex and ask to sit it out. The gaffer was always willing to listen, but he'd talk me into going. The FA were cracking down on all that anyway. There was a time when players would pull out of squads due to 'injury', but by then the associations were making us travel and would insist on medicals. It sounds mad that I would want to pull out, this is your country and it's an honour and all that, but such was the lack of faith or opportunity, I felt there were times when it was tiring and, without wanting to sound harsh, not worth it.

You trained, you played, you left. It could be a chore. The dressing room wasn't as close as at all our clubs and the media intrusion was insane. It will shock some England fans, but you could see that plenty of players couldn't wait to get the games done and go home.

That's why I like the current England set-up. I love Gareth Southgate's style. Gareth was around when I was and he would have seen those cliques. I was in one. Us United players would eat together and then all leave before everyone had finished their food. That's not right. I can see that now. Spain didn't become successful until they sorted out the relationship between the Real Madrid players and their Barcelona counterparts, and Gareth has put an end to all that now. The squad is unified and that's something my generation couldn't always say.

I hope today's gifted young players can bring the country the success we all want. There are so many exceptional youngsters coming through, and so why not? The environment is right, St George's is a great facility and the management is flexible enough to pick the right players, on form, at the right time, in the right position.

For me, that wasn't the case. I look back on my career with frustration and a sense that it was ultimately incomplete. I don't think I was entitled to a better England career, but I do wish I had been given more chances to prove myself. Instead, I was left in the pavilion. You could say, four managerial reigns stopped play.

9

FRIENDS AND ENEMIES

The time is right. Let's have it. I am fuming. Fuming! For months we haven't said a word to each other. He isn't my bag and everyone knows it, but we've got on with things. Now, though, Teddy Sheringham is saying his bit. I tell you, it is about to go off.

We were walking through the darkness of the Old Trafford tunnel, towards the dressing room. Heads bowed, shoulders hunched. It is February 1998 and the team have played out a disappointing 1–1 draw with Bolton Wanderers, a result that followed two successive league defeats, and the mood is glum.

Teddy, several yards further up from me, turned around, looked me in the eyes and growled, 'Their goal was your fault.'

His words hang in the air. What? I scored the equaliser, and now he's saying that!

As I say, the time is right. Let's have it.

I run up the tunnel and just as he gets to the dressing room, I'm ready to steam in. I'm screaming all sorts and trying to throw punches, but everyone's on me, stopping me, pulling us apart. The next thing I know, Roy Keane has me up against the wall and he's shouting in my face. 'What the **** are you doing, Coley? Sort yourself out. We're a team, Coley.' Blah, blah, blah. I'm not hearing him, but I calm down, and suddenly Roy is going for Teddy, ripping into him, and it's our turn to try to pull them apart.

'What's all that about, Skip?' I ask a clearly incensed Keane.

'You wanting to fight him reminded me of what a ***** he was to me at Nottingham Forest!'

That's football for you. The feud between me and Teddy would become well documented, but Roy's meltdown goes to show that bad blood within the game is more than common. Players move around, arguments go unsettled and memories are long. Conflicts, friction, discord, call it what you like, but in professional football, rivalries are everywhere.

Opposing players, team-mates, other managers, other clubs – all might be out to get you, whether it's to take your place in a team or the trophies you hold. In the late 1990s, at Manchester United, the club who had put themselves on top of the game's tree, everyone was our rival, both at home and abroad.

I could take supposed rivalries in my stride because

my biggest rival was always me. My biggest battle was always in my head. I had little concern for what other people were doing or saying about me. During the 1996–97 season, plenty was being said but as my own worst critic, who cared?

England managers and certain people in the press might have got a rise out of me but that was because they were saying things from the safety of a newspaper, that's different, but in general no one in the game could ever be as critical about me as me. Looking back, I'd like to have been nicer to myself. Less harsh. The thing is, it was that self-criticism that had got me to where I was, so that's that.

Rivals were perceived to be everywhere. All you needed to do was pick up a newspaper. I obviously had rivals for a place in the England team. Alan Shearer, Les Ferdinand, Ian Wright, Michael Owen. I was driven to compete for a spot in the team, but never to the point where I would disrespect any of them. People want to make you rivals and, yes, there can be a distance, but all you have to do is get to know someone for all that to drop away.

Take Robbie Fowler. Robbie for me was the best natural finisher I ever saw. I thought I was decent, but when I trained with Robbie on international duty, I blew out my cheeks. This kid is special. This was England, though. He was Liverpool. I was Manchester

United. We didn't mingle, didn't get close. Rarely spoke. He didn't particularly like me, and I didn't particularly like him. All that changed when I joined Manchester City in 2005 and Robbie was there. We got to know each other and Robbie said, 'You know what, Coley, you're not the arrogant **** I thought you were.'

In many minds, Alan Shearer and I were clear rivals. Two No. 9s, two goalscorers. He must be the man standing in the way of my place in the national team and my place at the top of the goalscoring charts. He must keep me up at night. That's wasn't the case at all.

For starters, Alan and I were totally different players. As a classic No. 9, he loved attacking crosses, whereas I wasn't interested in a winger getting to the byline and dinking a ball to the back post, because what was I going to do with that? I had two brilliant wingers at Manchester United, but they got the ball in early and low, and my pace and movement would try to get me on the end of things.

I had only respect for Alan, and in fact I am adamant that we could have played in the same team. We never got a run of games together for England, but as we were so different, I think we could have been successful. That's one of the reasons, in the summer of 1996, I wasn't too bothered when Manchester United were rumoured to be signing him from Blackburn.

It was all over the sports pages that the gaffer wanted

to take Alan, but being a United player, you get used to all that. Bring it on. I have never shirked a challenge, and persuading the gaffer to play us both would have been just that. Also, if the club choose to sell you, you're sad but that's the game and the next challenge is just around the corner.

The following year, Manchester United were heavily linked in the Saturday papers with a move for the Chilean striker Marcelo Salas. That afternoon, I scored a first-half hat-trick. I'm not saying I went out to prove myself, but there was never any point in worrying or sulking. It happened all the time. Not a problem.

In the end, Alan chose to go to Newcastle. To be honest, him coming to Old Trafford was a big ask, as he hated Manchester United and his hometown club was always going to be the dream move for him, so instead the gaffer went with a far less showbiz signing in a young Norwegian striker called Ole Gunnar Solskjaer.

None of us had heard of Ole. Who is this quiet, baby-faced guy? The £1.5 million the club had given Molde for his services seemed a lot of money too, but when we trained with him for the first time you could see the doubts fading away. Sharp. Super sharp. Great finisher with both feet, and we all stood back and took notice.

This being a group of footballers, I was ready for some stick and the lads didn't disappoint.

'Oh, Coley, that's you out, then.'

'Nice knowing you, Coley.'

'Got any plans, Saturday, Coley?'

'Don't worry, Coley, you look good in a tracksuit.'

You can always trust footballers to find humour in a team-mate's concerns. I can't imagine many nine-to-five jobs where people would laugh at the prospect of a colleague losing their job, but that's part of the fun. It's what makes us tick, it makes every day different, and as Ole slammed ball after ball into the corner of the net, I laughed along at their jibes.

The reality was, I got on with Ole from the start. He was refreshing. Loved to talk about football, and the art of finishing. We'd practise together and were similar. We would talk about the 'picture' we saw. That's the picture a striker will have in his head when a chance comes along. It's a snapshot, but it's vital and most finishers have it.

We would bounce things off each other. We actually played a lot together and ultimately pushed each other along. You have to see the whole team. Sure, Ole might have played instead of me, and I might have played in front of him, but you have to help the team or you are nothing. It has to be that way, because it's hard enough taking on opponents.

*

The 1996–97 Premier League campaign saw our rivals come from familiar places. Newcastle would once again give it a good go, Liverpool were also a threat for long periods and a new-look Arsenal were showing signs of life. We eventually strolled to the title, but there were times when things looked more than dodgy.

Unbeaten in our first nine games, we lost the next three autumn in a row. Luckily I missed them all! The first was a 5–0 defeat at Newcastle. A mad result, especially as we always used to do so well at St James'. I was on a train coming home from London. The train manager had spotted me and said, 'Have you seen the score?'

This was before smartphones, and so, no, I hadn't.

'Your lot are three down,' he said with a smile.

I thought he was just a Liverpool or City fan mugging me off until I got home, turned on the telly and caught the last couple of minutes. We'd lost 5–0 and I remember feeling sorry for the lads as they headed down the tunnel, towards the dressing room and what would have been a, let's say, disappointed gaffer.

On that occasion, the lads told me he went mad, but that wasn't always the case, and not every defeat was met with the fabled hairdryer. The gaffer was clever. I was on the end of some severe rants – my God, he could let me have it – but he picked his moments.

The following week we lost at Southampton, 6–3.

No blaming the colour of the shirts this time. Then there was a home defeat to Chelsea. Three consecutive defeats just didn't happen, but there was no panic.

The gaffer used to look at the big picture. Look at the manner of the defeats, give the opposition credit, praise our effort if our effort had been acceptable. Lay into our effort if it hadn't. The key thing was always to look forward, never to dwell on things, and even after that poor run, the instruction was to get back on the horse. There was always another big game around the corner and that was the biggest thing. It was the same with victories, by the way. Pats on the back, like bad bollockings, were short and sharp. Well done, but on we go.

I was 'fortunate' to miss those defeats due to a nasty injury I had picked up at Anfield in a supposedly run-of-the-mill reserve game. I'd had a bout of pneumonia in the summer and was working my way back to fitness. The gaffer thought a reserve game at Liverpool would help, but instead Neil Ruddock broke my ankle with a naughty tackle.

I had got in behind him and was in and was met with a crude lunge. I felt something go. I thought I could run it off, but it wasn't happening. Two fractured ankles. Ruddock never apologised, but that's not a problem.

The problem I had with it was later, when he went public saying he did it on purpose. He even said he did it because he's a good mate of Teddy Sheringham's and had set out to hurt me.

That's laughable, and he later took it back, but I had no time for someone like that. This was a reserve game, we were coming back from injury and illness and there was no need for it, but there it was. It was a major setback. My form and fitness at United hadn't been exactly where I wanted it to be. We'd won the Double but I knew I had to be better and now, as I started my recovery from this new injury, I realised my time was limited.

It was during that recovery that I really focused. Mentally, I battered myself, telling myself that this was it, this was the time, this was my moment. I had to come back stronger and sharper. I had to be a better all-round player, fitter and even more committed. It worked. The head space that injury gave me was key to my progress. I worked my socks off getting back, and from there I came back the Manchester United player I had always wanted to be. Thanks, Razor.

In that 1996–97 season, for long spells Ruddock's Liverpool looked like being our main challengers for the Premier League. Top of the league at Christmas and into January, Roy Evans's team, thanks mainly to the brilliant young Robbie Fowler, looked like ending their seven-year wait for the title.

I had arrived in Manchester knowing about the rivalry with Liverpool from the outside, but I didn't fully get just how intense it was. It took an evening with Giggsy to make me understand. I hadn't been at the club long when Ryan and I decided on a night out. The gaffer has spies all over Manchester, so Giggsy suggested going to Liverpool for a night at Cream, a well-known club.

On the way we met up with a few guys, who I presumed were his mates. These lads were big. Huge. It didn't take me long to realise that they were our security for the night. Cream was a great night out, lots of the lads would go, but we were always protected by these fellas. They would follow us to the bar, the toilets, everywhere we went. I never felt threatened by anyone, but the presence of these lads was telling.

On the pitch, we went to Anfield in April, having knocked our rivals from top spot and knowing a win would effectively end their title hopes. I absolutely loved playing at Anfield. I had scored there on my first visit with Newcastle in 1994, and there was something about the place – the buzz from the crowd, the intensity of the fixture, the history, the short coach journey, the winding streets approaching the ground. I loved it and it showed in my record there.

I got eleven goals at Liverpool in my career, more than any other away ground. The crowd was so tight to us, the away section behind a goal rather than up in the gods. Our fans were always so loud there, adding to the atmosphere. It got my juices flowing every time and the goals would follow.

It takes me back to my time as a youth-team player at Arsenal. Pat Rice always said I did much better when I was angry. 'Get Coley angry and the defenders are in trouble,' he'd say. He was right. The needle involved in the Liverpool fixture, especially at Anfield, got my tail up, and I rarely had a quiet game.

The gaffer knew it. I could have gone twenty games without a goal, I could be carrying an injury, but when the Anfield game came around, I'd be playing. There was never much of a team talk at Anfield, the occasion spoke for itself, and that day we went out and played very well. Gary Pallister got two and I got a late goal to settle it. Liverpool were gone and we went on to retain our title.

Every league title was met with huge celebration. It was always the gaffer's priority. 'Be the best at the end of the season' was always the shout. Europe, though, so ingrained in the fabric of the football club, was always a massive ambition, and that season we all felt we had a great chance of winning the Champions League.

It wouldn't be easy. Juventus, the strongest team around, became almost a rival in the late 1990s, so many times did we play them. I loved the challenge they presented and, as a striker, tried to learn every time I went up against them. Talk about an eye-opener.

First of all, there were the little dirty tricks. The sly punches, the pinching, the shirt-pulling. You had to keep your cool because lose your rag in Europe and you were off. Then there was just how tightly you were marked. In the Premier League, defenders might mark you at arm's length, covering the chance of you spinning in behind them. When I played against Juventus, they had such trust in their team-mates to cover any such run, that they would mark tightly, and space was always such a premium. When they were on it, it was like facing a wall. You couldn't break them down.

What a battle it always was, but I relished it. They were so knowledgeable, so streetwise, it became a battle of body *and* mind. Chances were hard to come by and if one came along, bang, you'd better put it away. It was funny. In the Premier League, if you missed one, the lads were all shouting, 'Head up, Coley, keep going, mate, next one.' Not in the Champions League, not against Juventus.

I missed one in Turin once. Roy was all over me, giving me stick, but then I heard Gary Neville. Yes, Gary Neville! 'For ***** sake, Coley, stick it in the

******* net!' I had to smile. 'All right, Nev, I'm not trying to miss.' All you got back was daggers from everyone.

You couldn't blame them. When you're facing the attacking threat Juventus carried then, you want any sort of respite. There were times when you just wanted to stand back and admire the grace of Zinedine Zidane. He was that good. The gaffer would never bother coming up with some masterplan to stop him, though. What was the point? Asking Keane to do a job on him was a waste of Roy's talent and it might not even work.

Then there were all the other players they had. Alessandro Del Piero was some player, who would punish any space you gave him, and there was Alen Bokšić from Croatia. We called him Roadrunner. My God, he was quick. I remember a goal he scored against us out there. I can see Butty running through treacle trying to stop him as he sprinted onto a Zidane pass. Poor Butty had no chance.

I look back and smile at the football pitches I shared with some of the game's true greats. The 1990s were a golden period. Today we talk of Lionel Messi and Cristiano Ronaldo, and of course they are among the best ever, but back then there was a selection of footballers all vying for top spot. The Brazilian Ronaldo, Rivaldo, Zidane, Del Piero, Luís Figo, Paolo Maldini. I could go on. I have plenty of medals, but I often take more pleasure from the names I played with and against. I'd come a long way from a kid most people thought would end up behind bars.

Hopes of a Champions League final against Juventus were dashed on a night at Old Trafford in April 1997 that still makes me feel gutted, over twenty years later. How we didn't beat Borussia Dortmund in the semi-final, I still don't know. It still annoys me.

We absolutely pulverised them. We had lost 1–0 out there and wondered how, but we were confident we could overturn that at our place. I can't explain what happened. We'd battered Porto in the quarters and set about the Germans in the same fashion, but we couldn't take our chances. It wasn't to be, and in the end Dortmund even won the match, 1–0.

It was agonising. The dressing room was a morgue. The gaffer was so low. He had felt this was his chance. He wanted to take on the best and Marcello Lippi's Juventus awaited. There were plenty of times when we won football matches and our opponents must have wondered how, so it works both ways, but we all left Old Trafford that night gutted that a real chance to progress had gone.

Eric Cantona was mortified. So much so that he retired. I'm not saying that game was the sole reason, but I do think he felt that if we couldn't win the trophy he so coveted that season, maybe we never would. Not long after the season ended, he announced his retirement and he was gone. There wasn't even a goodbye, but that's football.

Towards the end of the season, I lost my grandfather, Vincent. He'd been such a vibrant, strong and loving part of the life of me and my family, his going was a huge blow to me and one I didn't handle well. My grandmother had died six months earlier and we tried to rally around him, but they were soul partners and you could see him drifting away. I sincerely believe he died of a broken heart.

I have never been good at talking about or dealing with death and grief. I would have to face my own mortality years later, but back then I suppressed everything, choosing to look out for my mum, to focus on her. I kept my grief locked away and I know that it had an adverse effect on my whole life. It was over twenty years ago, but the pain of losing him is still very real.

No one could replace my grandfather, but at Old Trafford the talk was all about who would replace Eric. One day in pre-season training that summer, Giggsy and I were in the showers discussing just that. A few names were mentioned but we both agreed on Matt Le Tissier. We rated the Southampton man very highly. He was different from Eric but he had a similar way about him. He was his own man, he had that swagger and we felt he could have the same effect as the Frenchman.

A few days later I was at home with Shirley and the news came on. 'Teddy Sheringham has signed for Manchester United.' My jaw dropped. It was a comedy moment. 'You ******* what?' I shouted at the TV. My head was spinning. The gaffer had no idea about my feelings for Teddy, and why would that bother him anyway, but I was ready for the lads to have their say. Once again, no one let me down.

'Your best mate is on his way, Coley.'

'You must be well pleased, Coley.'

'Got a new room-mate, Coley?'

It's funny. Any fault, any little concern in football, they are always picked on and used as humour. You have to laugh. You also have to get on with things. Teddy knew how I felt and didn't try to build bridges but again, why should he? We muddled along but it was bad. We never spoke. After our bust-up in the tunnel, the gaffer called us into his office like naughty schoolboys and told us to sort things out: he couldn't condone fighting in the team. As Manchester United players, it had better stop.

We nodded and said the right things to the gaffer,

but we never sorted it out. It was always there. The incident in the tunnel proved it could go off at any time. We were volatile men and any wrong word might spark another bust-up. It got so bad that when Dwight Yorke signed later in 1998, he would pass on messages from us. 'Yorkey,' Teddy would say. 'Ask Coley X, Y or Z.' Dwight would turn to me and ask me the question and I'd reply to him, and he would pass on the answer to Teddy.

Feuds in the dressing room were nothing compared to a new rivalry brewing in the Premier League. Arsenal had improved since their new manager, Arsène Wenger, had arrived in 1996 and now they were ready to make serious inroads up the table.

There had been a long-standing dislike between the clubs. I had been a youth-team player at Arsenal when the two senior teams clashed at Old Trafford in 1990. That had lingered. One of my first games against Arsenal for Manchester United had opened my eyes further. Steve Bruce and Ian Wright were going for it. Tackles, elbows, words said. Brucie left it on him and put him in the front row of seats and Wrighty had had enough. 'See you at half-time,' he shouted.

You hear that a lot, but then as we walked up the tunnel (what is it about that tunnel?) it all went off.

Wrighty lost it and cracked our captain in the face. Cue bedlam. These are your team-mates and so you join in, but I was thinking, 'Bloody hell, is this what goes on?'

That intensity never waned, it only became more acute, a mixture of going for the same honours and, frankly, a dislike of certain individuals. That seemed to be how it was between Roy Keane and Arsenal's new midfield general, Patrick Vieira.

I think there was actually respect between them. I'm sure Pat respected Schiz (my nickname for Roy, and one I somehow got away with), but Schiz was ice-cool. You just knew he was going to go out there and give it his absolute all. He didn't give a toss about who he was up against, but because the challenge against Pat was that bit harder, he relished it.

As his team-mate, you knew what was about to happen and you knew how important Roy would be to the match. The midfield was key. The game could be won or lost depending on who came out on top between Roy and Pat. If Roy plays his game and does his job, we're good to go. So often he did. What great games they were. The sort of matches you can't stand to miss.

Arsenal came to Old Trafford in March 1998 and won 1–0, thanks to a Marc Overmars goal. It was a massive blow and one that helped secure the Londoners an unlikely title. The hunters had become the hunted. Arsenal chased us down and, thanks to our threadbare squad, the result of serious injuries to serious players, Arsenal were simply too good.

Denis Irwin's stability and assurance had been missing since October and Roy Keane had been out since September. Roy had done his ligaments against Leeds in an infamous incident at Elland Road. Roy was challenging Alf Inge Haaland, a player he had little time for, but his studs got caught in the turf and his knee went. The Norwegian took offence at the challenge, and while Roy was in agony on the ground, he leant down and shouted some abuse about cheating in his face.

I was quickly on the scene, checking on Roy, and his eyes told me a line had been crossed. He had this steely look. His ligaments were in absolute bits and the pain he was in must have been severe, but he had other things on his mind. Revenge. 'No **** is going to stand over me and call me a cheat,' he said. You could tell he wasn't joking.

Sure enough, three and a half years later, Haaland came to Old Trafford with Manchester City and, crack, Roy did his knee. Like a Sicilian hitman, Schiz had carried out his vendetta. I'm not saying what he did was right, and I certainly don't think he set out to seriously injure the player, in fact Roy has said just that, but rivals were rivals. Today he would have been banned for a season, but back then he operated just within the, let's say, more relaxed limits.

Without our captain, and several other players, the 1997–98 season had become a slog. Arsenal took advantage and in Europe we also ran out of steam. I had got a hat-trick at Feyenoord in the group stages, which I was very proud of. Three goals away from home in the Champions League is an achievement, whoever the opposition, but the night was soured by Denis Irwin's knee injury, the fact that our fans were attacked in the stands and, less seriously, David May's hilarious (Maysie was one of the funniest man I ever met!) meltdown when he was followed all over the stadium by a hapless drug-tester wanting a sample.

We faced Monaco in the quarter-finals and were again left wondering how we managed to lose. Though we were not as dominant as the previous year, we still expected to beat Monaco, but we were undone by a wonder strike from David Trezeguet. Once again, we'd fallen short in Europe.

It was to prove a difficult summer. On one hand, I was pleased with my form. I had worked hard and felt my overall game was much better. The punters, always so supportive towards me, voted me their player of the year, and any self-doubts about my place in the team had long gone.

What I couldn't shake was the pure disappointment at losing our title to Arsenal and being knocked out of Europe by Monaco. Arsenal played their last league game at home to Everton. It was a party at Highbury and I forced myself to watch every minute. I say forced because it was hell. Tony Adams scored a great goal at the end and stood, his arms wide, taking the applause.

I love Tony but as he lifted the Premier League Trophy, I was gutted. I couldn't turn the TV off, though. That was our trophy he was lifting and I wanted it back. I sat there, cringing, but it was adding fuel to my fire. I was in a mood all summer. A proper monk on. Usually you want to get away, lie by a pool, recharge, but all I could think about was Monaco knocking us out, and Tony with our trophy.

Two words stayed with me all summer. Next season. Next season.

10

PROMISED LAND

It is all so familiar. The setting: Old Trafford. Our old place of work. A celebration to mark the twenty years that have passed since Manchester United won the Treble. Familiar walls, familiar faces. The same jokes as laughter fills the room. The smiles are as wide as some of the newly stretched waistlines.

The gaffer walks in. Silence. The spring in his step belies his seventy-seven years. The twinkle in his eye mocks any recent health concerns. Like an old head-master standing in front if his favourite old class, he is full of life and begins to talk. He tells us how lovely it is to be with us all again and what a pleasure it was to manage us that season. His eyes misting up, he pauses, looks around and says, 'Bloody hell, Henning, remember your clearance off the line against Inter, here?'

That's what I love about the 1998–99 season. There are so many iconic moments to replay in the mind or share again with those who want to. Ole's late winner against Liverpool in the FA Cup, Roy's header in Turin, Peter's penalty save at Villa Park, Giggsy's celebration moments later, Teddy's equaliser followed by Ole's winner in Barcelona. All are poster moments for a never-forgotten season, but there was so much more.

A whole squad together, fighting on three fronts. There were plenty of less celebrated moments that are instantly memorable when called upon by the mind's eye. Two decades on, the gaffer only had to mention Henning Berg's brilliantly athletic denial of a clear Inter Milan opportunity to score a decisive away goal in the quarter-final of the Champions League and immediately we were all right there, together.

Everyone at the football club that season can say they won the Treble. Everyone made a contribution. From the punters who came everywhere in massive numbers, to the laundry ladies who always met us players with a smile, the whole club were swept along on this incredible wave as we made history.

The thing is, two months into the season, I felt anything but part of something special. In fact, I'd go as far as saying that I had been totally kiboshed. The gaffer had four strikers and I was very much fourth on that list. There were times when Giggsy and Scholesy played up top in front of me and, yes, I wondered just how long I'd be around the place.

At Manchester United you become more than used

to speculation. Having missed out on silverware the previous season, the gaffer was after a new strike force and the papers were full of talk about who might come in. Patrick Kluivert's name was mentioned and I'm sure the club were very serious about getting him.

Fergie wanted two, though, and the pursuit of Aston Villa's Dwight Yorke was real too, so much so that the club paid a massive £12.5 million for his exciting services. With the Kluivert talk not going away, it seemed that someone would have to. Ole was happy to stay and play games when asked; Teddy was a bit frustrated too, I think; and I got the impression that any cash raised from selling me would help fund a move for Kluivert.

It was a bit awkward but, as I have said, that's football and you embrace whatever new challenge awaits you. There was some vague talk about me being part of the move for Dwight and going to Villa, but it never amounted to anything. In the end, nor did the gaffer's moves for Kluivert and so the season began with four of us waiting for the nod.

Dwight wouldn't have to wait long. It was clear that he was the gaffer's main man. A brilliant footballer who gave the gaffer the movement, skill and goalscoring ability he desired was clearly going to start, but who would partner him? Not me. Not at first.

I had played in the Charity Shield, a game we lost

3–0 to Arsenal, and that result was replicated when the team went to Highbury in late September. Only I wasn't involved at all this time. I hadn't been playing for the first games of the season, and the gaffer had asked me to play in the reserves. I wasn't having it. I was twenty-seven, my peak, and being asked to play stiff football wasn't going to make me smile. Not being involved, watching Teddy and Ole play games with Yorkey – it was doing my head in, and I told the gaffer that I wasn't turning out for the reserves.

'Fair enough, but don't bother bringing your boots to Arsenal.'

I was frustrated and desperate to play, but I wasn't sulking. People might have had the perception that, with Dwight's arrival, I was throwing my toys out of the pram, but that is untrue. I welcomed Dwight with open arms, a new team-mate who became a best mate. I took him out, had him over for dinner, showed him the best places to buy a house; there was an instant friendship.

It was the same with all the new signings (Teddy being the exception). Quite recently, I bumped into Ruud van Nistelrooy and he wanted to thank me for making his arrival so smooth and helping him settle in. I might have this image from the outside that I would be sulky and make trouble, but all I cared about was United improving and the team having success. I always felt I could be part of that success, and I'd work hard to be just that, but a new striker arriving, I'd do anything to help them.

One player who needed some extra help that summer was David Beckham. After he'd been sent off in the World Cup defeat to Argentina, the knives were out. The abuse Becks took in the papers was disgraceful. They went for him. It was vicious, and of course much of the footballing public followed suit. We went to West Ham early in the season, and it was vile.

The press knew that anything to do with Becks sold newspapers. He has a mum, a dad, sisters, a family? So what? Cue a load of nasty headlines and the country had their scapegoat. Plenty doubted how a young man would react, but the club rallied around him. He'd been there since he was a boy and had a steely nerve not yet seen. We all knew about his work ethic, but the way he dealt with all that hate, I was impressed.

I was also excited with the new signings. Jesper Blomqvist was a skilful addition and Jaap Stam, a player I hadn't heard of, immediately showed his qualities in training. A few of us wondered if he really was Dutch. The footballers from Holland we'd previously encountered could be quite arrogant, letting you know they know it all and have seen it all. Not Jaap. He was eager to listen and learn and had no doubts that life in the Premier League wasn't going to be easy.

That summer, Roy Keane was like a new signing. He

had worked like a Trojan to get back from his nasty knee injury and he came back faster than most players could and looked strong. We'd missed his presence and drive, and when he returned he was lean and had this look in his eye. Schiz meant business.

Our first league game was against Leicester at Old Trafford, and after seventy-six minutes, it was clear our visitors meant business too. We were 2–0 down, Jaap Stam was learning that centre-forwards like Emile Heskey can put it about a bit and the team were staring an early setback in the face. But we found a late surge that would define a season. Teddy got one and an injury-time free-kick from Becks (or Superstar as I now called him) salvaged a point.

It was a stodgy start to the season. Both for the team and for me. After another draw and a couple of wins, that defeat at Arsenal left us tenth in the division. After my punishment at Highbury I was back on the bench for the midweek visit of Liverpool to Old Trafford. I got on and felt sharp, beating Phil Babb to set up Scholesy for a brilliant goal. Maybe the gaffer saw a spark there, because for the next fixture, at Southampton, I was given a start. It was a game that changed everything.

The team won 3–0 but it was the nature of that win.

Yorkey and I clicked straight away. It was so much fun from the off and the team picked up on it. People watching that day must have thought that the gaffer was a genius, having us work together in training, before unleashing us in October. The gaffer was a genius but not on this occasion. He knows it, we know it. The partnership was stumbled upon. There was no grand plan. In fact, I was in no one's plans!

We didn't even train together. The club wasn't big on doing interplay or phases of play in training; we weren't even in the same small-sided games, as we did England v the rest of the world. We might have done a bit of finishing together with Ole, but I don't think I ever passed Dwight a ball in training.

It was so off the cuff. On ten minutes I made a run to the left-hand touchline, but I instinctively knew that he would be filling the space I left, and I crossed a low ball in for Yorkey to score. From there it was pure joy.

It was so natural. Everything built on trust, believing that we were making the right moves for each other and therefore the team. Thinking about it brings a smile to my face today. It was a friendship that worked on the pitch as well as off it. I didn't get on with Teddy yet we played well together, but now I had a real mate, one who never stopped smiling, and it was magic.

I remember at the time, I likened meeting Yorkey to meeting a beautiful woman and starting a perfect relationship. In so many ways we were chalk and cheese. Dwight was all collars up and flamboyance. Loud clothes on, loving the camera, straight to the front of a queue. I am happy to sit in the shadows, avoiding the limelight. Reserved.

He had that constant smile. People would say I was always frowning, but next to Yorkey, everyone is always frowning! I was the organised one. He was my wake-up call, every morning phoning me to ask what time he had to be in for training. For all those differences, we never had a cross word, and to this day we've never had one. In fact, sometimes all I have to do is look at Dwight and he knows what I'm saying and we crack up.

When he arrived, Yorkey was single. Very single. He was a boy. I'd go out with him, and try to be a decent wingman, and it got me in trouble. One Sunday I was in the papers. A kiss-and-tell. The actual story was full of rubbish, but there you go, the fact was I had been silly. I was old enough to know better and my private life was going to get very hard.

After the Southampton game, you could see in the gaffer's face that he thought ours was a partnership that could drive the team forward. I felt good, I was scoring and playing well, and the team were improving. It did make me laugh, though, that whenever people talked about my game, it was always in relation to other players, and who I was playing with.

'Will Cole be able to dovetail with Cantona?' and 'He looks better with Sheringham,' and then 'Look at his game now that Yorke is there.' It was years later that I realised there was an agenda with me and the media. The 'he needs loads of chances' line had been jumped on by some, and now it was all about who I played with. No one praised Teddy because of the partners he had. Alan Shearer was simply a great striker; it didn't matter who he partnered. I was working my socks off to improve and it was paying off, but there it was, someone else was clearly making me better. As I say, agendas.

The gaffer would tell the team, 'Just get the ball to the forwards, and let them get on with it. They'll win us the game.' That wasn't true, but we did play with a pace – don't over-pass (the gaffer went mad if we over-passed), get the ball in the opposition's last third and chances will come. Becks and Giggsy were superb all season, their delivery always early and right on the mark. Everything was good.

We did have a tiny blip in December, going out of the League Cup at Spurs and losing at home to Middlesbrough. It coincided with the news that Peter Schmeichel would leave us at the end of the season and that Brian Kidd, the gaffer's brilliant assistant, was leaving immediately, to take the Blackburn job.

Peter was going to be a huge loss but that was fine, we could hope he'd go out on a high, but Kiddo leaving, that was more unsettling. For me personally, he'd been a tremendous help when I arrived, working with me on my overall game and helping me improve. The lads loved him.

We used to call him Capello. He used to travel to AC Milan a lot, observe and come back with a load of great ideas. There were no fitness trainers then, no analysts, just Kiddo sorting things out. He took pre-season every summer, did all the sessions, and they were always fresh, innovative, exciting – and that, let me tell you, is not always the case in football.

We understood that he had ambitions to be a boss in his own right, but we were going to miss him and his methods. The gaffer, too, but he was in no rush to appoint someone straight away, not when he had Jim Ryan around, an experienced coach at the club and, again, a very popular figure. We called him 'Dunga' because in our games, he would sit in the midfield, spraying the ball about like the Brazilian World Cup-winning captain. Dunga had an old classic Ferrari and wouldn't stop going on about it, how he had fixed something on it, how he had bought something new for it, how he was taking it out on Friday.

He was a top man, but too often sounded more like *Top Gear*.

I used to sit and talk a lot to Jim, and with Brian McClair. Choccy, as he was known, was another great presence at the club, a wealth of knowledge and experience, able to give sound advice, helping us players become better pros and people. That was important at Manchester United and, as I said earlier, the success we shared was down to so many more people than you could see on the surface.

I used to love the laundry ladies. I could walk into the laundry room and have a cup of tea, always share a laugh and walk out feeling more chilled. These are the people who stay at a club, make a training ground tick, take the pressure off by just being themselves. I always thought, me and the boys might get all the plaudits, but their role was vital because they brought normality and would tell us when we were being prats. The ladies recently left the club and I got myself to Carrington, the training ground, to say goodbye. We shared a cuppa and the usual jokes and I was touched to see they had a picture of me up in the room.

Washing away the stains from our small blip was the gaffer. He had missed the Middlesbrough defeat for family reasons and on his return he called a meeting. We'd drawn a few games, shipped a few goals and losing to 'Boro just wasn't on. There was no big blow-out, though. Just a quiet word. 'Let's stop with all the sloppy goals, shall we?' We didn't lose another game all season.

The gaffer was brilliantly simple. Hated gimmicks. We'd laugh at times when he tried to use the magnet board, struggling to move the magnets around before giving up. 'Stuff that. Coley, just get in the box.' There was no need for grand gestures or big tactical lectures. That season he'd decided to scrap the videos of the opposition. Too often you would be shown clips of your opponents' best bits and you'd leave the room thinking you were playing Brazil's 1970 World Cup-winning team.

That all went and as 1998 became 1999, the team talk before the Premier League matches was mainly just 'You're all looking great, you look strong, form is great, play like you have been and you'll win. Now go and enjoy yourself.' You might get a bit about set plays, but even then it was 'Pick up your man and stay with your man'. Zonal marking? Don't be silly, that was a nonsense to him.

Europe was not much different. The gaffer appreciated the strengths of the coaches and the players we had to face and might look at things from more of a tactical stance, but not once did we ever go anywhere without the sole purpose of winning. In the Champions League we were drawn in what was called the 'Group of Death', as we would play Barcelona and Bayern Munich, as well as Brondby, but we knew and the gaffer knew we could get at teams, that we had players they would fear too.

I loved those games. Our approach was a dream for strikers because we were on the front foot. We drew our first games at home to Barcelona and then away in Munich. Both close, well-fought games, and the eleven goals we put past Brondby in the next two clashes meant we were in an OK place going into the last two games. Barcelona away had some history for the club, having been beaten there 4–0 in 1994, and we went there fully committed to victory.

We got a more-than-decent 3–3 draw but we had attacked to win. Yorkey had equalised after their early opener and I got us 2–1 up with a second-half effort. Man, I loved that goal. I can watch it today and it seems to get better; it epitomises the way Dwight and I were working together. Keane fizzed it in, Dwight stepped over it, we played a one-two and I was in, a quick picture in my head of what I wanted to do, and the ball was nestled in the Barcelona net.

The celebrations were memorable too. The night before we had trained at the Nou Camp and, typically, I was just ticking over, not wanting to exert myself too much. The gaffer was watching and was on me. 'Coley, focus!' OK, boss, yes, boss, no problem, boss. But that was the shout for the rest of the session; 'FOCUS!'

To the side of that goal, by the corner flag, there was an advertising board, for the Ford Focus. I said to the lads that if I scored, I'd run over to it. 'Yeah, OK, Coley,' they said, and then when it happened, that's just what I did. FOCUS!

We ended up drawing the game 3–3 and went through thanks to a 1–1 draw at home to Bayern Munich. We were in the quarters and we could *focus* on the league and the start of the FA Cup. We impressed with a 6–2 win at Leicester in the league and beat Middlesbrough in the FA Cup, and then drew Liverpool at Old Trafford in the fourth round. That would be juicy.

Michael Owen's early goal looked to have won them the tie, but we just didn't stop. Yorkey got a late equaliser before Ole's last-gasp winner. That was so sweet. It summed us up as a team. We used to say, 'We don't lose games, we just run out of time.'

It was part of the very fabric of the place. When I first joined it was a matter of weeks before I knew what it was to be a Manchester United player. There are the standards set, but there is also a mentality and a personality. The latter is all about the style of play, while the mentality is looking out for each other, making sure opponents never take liberties, but also never giving up. The whole squad understood that.

The gaffer was a big part of that too. Great managers can get their teams playing the game in their personality and we would all play as if him. He had that never-say-die attitude himself and it transmitted itself to the players. It helped him that we were a self-motivating bunch of men, and if standards dropped, he had a captain like Roy Keane, who would come down hard on anyone he felt wasn't getting it.

I was never on the end of one of Roy's rants, but they were always tasty, and if an individual wasn't on the end of one, the whole team was. The gaffer could just stand back and let him go to town on us all, before saying a few calmer words, knowing his captain had done the heavy lifting. They were very similar and maybe that explains why they eventually fell out.

Roy had a lot of freedom to do the gaffer's work, but maybe towards the end that freedom was too much. The power afforded Roy was probably what did for him in the end. In the Treble season, though, Roy's input was incredible. All he wanted was the best for his team and he drove us on as if possessed.

Ole certainly was possessed at Nottingham Forest, coming on as a late sub in January and scoring four goals in the last ten minutes in an emphatic 8–1 win.

An old friend from Nottingham, one of my elders, was in prison at the time and would send me letters. I always remember him writing to me and saying how annoyed I must have been that Ole had come on for me and got all those goals. Why would I worry about that? It always made me smile. People assume there is so much competition at football clubs, but there wasn't then.

I scored a big equaliser against Arsenal in our next game. We should have won the game, but by now we were top of the league and keeping our rivals at bay was vital. Especially as our Champions League commitments were on the horizon and a quarter-final clash with Inter Milan was looming.

The talk in the papers prior to the game was of David Beckham's 'reunion' with Diego Simeone, the Argentine midfielder he had clashed with when getting sent off for England at the World Cup. To us, it was no big deal, but the cameras were all focusing on the pre-match handshake. It was a lot of fuss about nothing and Becks was absolutely brilliant that night, the accuracy and venom of his crosses putting two goals on a plate for Yorkey to secure us a 2–0 win.

There were little moments. That Henning Berg goal-line clearance preventing their away goal, but I also remember Jaap, early on, being leant on by their centre-forward, Iván Zamorano. It was a setpiece and the Chilean striker was trying to muscle in. Jaap gave him a nice little dig, as if to say, 'Oi, this is our turf, behave yourself.' I remember thinking, 'That'll do.'

The second leg was going to be tough. Two-goal leads are one thing, but the San Siro is one of football's hardest places to go. Simeone was very loud in the tunnel before the game, rallying his troops, but that had no effect on us. We were a confident bunch and vocals weren't going to get them far. We knew we were in for a game, but we just felt we would score in every game we played.

Talking of scoring goals, Ronaldo, the original Ronaldo, would play that night. He had missed the first leg with an injury and it was clear he wasn't fully fit. His knee was bad and I'd guess he played at 40 per cent. All I can say is thank God for that. Ronaldo at less than half fitness was some player. Some of the things he did took the breath away, but we stood firm, and even under pressure we looked comfortable. You need a bit of luck to win any competition and Ronaldo's lack of fitness was fortunate, but with Henning having another brilliant game, we kept them at bay.

Well, for an hour. There was no panic, though, and with fifteen minutes left we levelled on the night through Scholesy, an away goal that killed the tie. Gary Neville had looped a typically high cross into the box and I cushioned it down with my head for Paul to do the rest. A few years earlier I would have headed for goal, but not now, and that is because of the work Kiddo had done with me. That initial chat we had had when I joined from Newcastle and him telling me that scoring forty-one goals wasn't enough at Old Trafford had always stayed with me, and with hard work, my appreciation of the players around me had got better and better. My assist record is actually very good and not talked about much. I'm very proud of it.

Games were coming thick and fast now. Players love that. I got two goals in a big 2–1 win at Newcastle in March to keep us top of the Premier League, and each game was met with excitement. No talk of trebles from us, of course, but what gets the juices flowing is the momentum we had. Momentum can be like an extra player, and winning becomes a habit. We had been losing at Newcastle, but it's like muscle memory: no panic, just the knowledge that we will win, just like last week.

You take nothing for granted, of course, the opponents are too good to do that, but in April there was nothing but a buzz about our dressing room as we prepared to play Arsenal in the semi-final of the FA Cup and Juventus in the semi-final of the Champions League. It gives me goosebumps just thinking about it.

The first Arsenal game was a tight 0–0. The star of

the show was the referee, David Elleray, who disallowed a Roy Keane goal for reasons only he knows. He was a housemaster at Harrow School and wasn't the easiest to communicate with. Roy absolutely hated him and a few fans felt the same way, especially later that season when he gave a very dubious penalty against us at Anfield before sending Denis Irwin off for doing nothing more than trying to keep the ball in play.

The replay proved to be one of the great nights in the club's and the FA Cup's history. I, though, wasn't involved. I had played the first game but I had a slight ankle knock. Don't worry about that, just strap it up and let's go. The gaffer had other ideas. 'No, you're not playing. We have bigger games coming up.'

He was talking about the Champions League semi-final second leg, and he might have been right, but I didn't see things that way. This was a cup semi-final against Arsenal, at Villa Park, brilliant, under flood-lights. I wasn't happy at being up in the stands.

Looking back, I guess I should be grateful for having such a good view of one of the great nights in English football. What a game! Becks had put us ahead, but Bergkamp equalised before having the chance to win it from the spot late on, after Phil Neville brought down Ray Parlour. '*Oh for **** sake, Phil, that's the treble ******!*' But Peter saved it and, despite Roy being sent off (by Elleray, of course), we were still in it and the game plan was to keep things simple and win a penalty shoot-out.

That's why, when Giggsy picked the ball up in the Arsenal half in extra-time, I started to say, 'Pass it.' He moved forward. 'Pass it.' He approached the penalty area. 'Pass it.' He dropped the shoulder and wriggled past Martin Keown and Lee Dixon, and now it was 'Shoot!' Giggsy smashed the ball and it was in the roof of the net.

Bedlam. We were off our seats, the bench was going crazy, fans were running on the pitch, Giggsy had his top off and was spinning it over his head and the game was won. That is what football is all about. The dressing room was on fire that night – the directors, players, staff, champagne. Each big win was pouring fuel on those flames as the buzz got bigger and better.

Prior to the Arsenal games, we had played Juventus at home in the first leg of the Champions League semi-final. It was a tough game. Zidane, of course, but Antonio Conte next to him in midfield, he was an absolute dog. Conte got their big away goal and we had to dig deep. It would be easy to succumb to feelings of inferiority, to tell yourself that there is no shame in losing to this mob, but you don't. You know you are there on merit, that you are their equals and, to be fair, we got at them in the second half and deserved our late Giggsy goal.

We were level, we could go to Turin knowing we had to not lose and we had a good chance. Eleven minutes in and we were 2–0 down and any game plan was out of the window. That's where the team spirit, the team ethic, kicks in again. There's a long way to go, any thoughts of self-pity must be killed; there is still a game to be won.

Even up against it in Turin, against Juventus, it was not hard to focus. As footballers, everything you have worked for is in front of you. At this level, you can always hope because you are in control. Punters struggle to see hope at 2–0 down, but players who train hard and have power to change things, they must drive forward. At United that was key.

When Roy rose to head in a Becks corner, we were right back in it. Roy Keane was incredible that night. Booked and missing the final, he dragged us up to a level that would win us the game. I know he took offence at the gaffer writing in his book that his performance was special in Turin, but I don't care. Sorry, Roy, but you were.

He said that you wouldn't praise a postman for delivering his letters, but I'm sorry, if a postman had to compete against the fiercest dogs on the street, and still delivered all the letters on time despite being bitten early on, then, yes, you would praise him.

Keane was an absolute joke that night. He was an

absolute joke most of the time, but that night, it was a different level. There was something wrong with him; in fact, there was something wrong with all of us. That night in Turin is the most special performance I have ever been involved in. It was a domino effect. Maybe it was started by the captain, but soon each player involved saw his team-mate's efforts and went up a gear himself.

Before half-time we were level. I, for some reason, found myself wide right. Becks cushioned a header for me and I controlled it with the sole of my boot, before getting my head up and seeing Yorkey peeling off his marker. They say a centre-forward knows what a centre-forward wants, it's just the technique that might be off, but the curling cross I produced . . . it was like David bloody Beckham!

Yorkey headed us level and the dressing room at half-time was absolutely buzzing. 'They've gone,' the gaffer kept saying. We were champing at the bit to get out there. 'They've gone.' We believed him. Let's go.

That forty-five minutes of football? I get emotional thinking about it, thinking about the effort each and every one of us put in, the togetherness, the sheer reluctance to leave that ground without a ticket to the Nou Camp for the final. We were possessed.

Juventus had chances, but Peter was brilliant in goal, as was the whole back four, and we were stretching

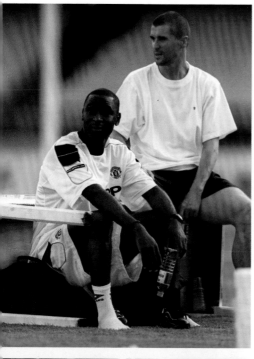

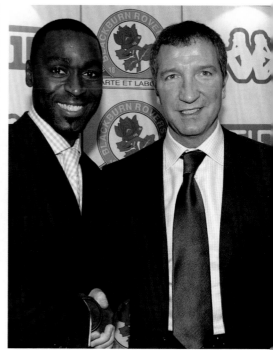

Above left: Sitting out training in Rio de Janeiro's fabled Maracanã Stadium in 2000 with Roy Keane – a class act.

Above right: I've just signed for Graeme Souness at Blackburn in 2001, blissfully unaware of the problems ahead.

Left: Celebrating scoring the winning goal in the the 2002 League Cup final.

Below: Rapture and relief are etched upon my face after what was the pinnacle of my career at Blackburn Rovers.

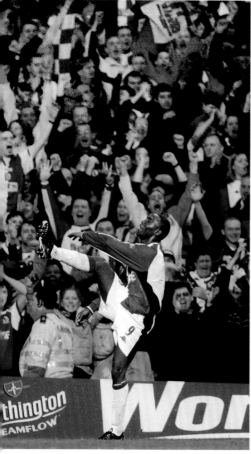

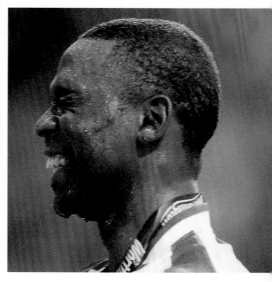

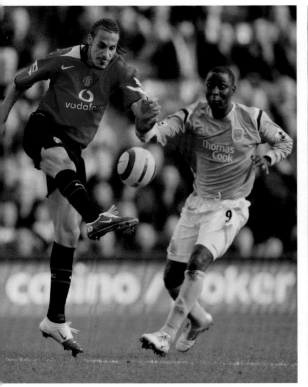

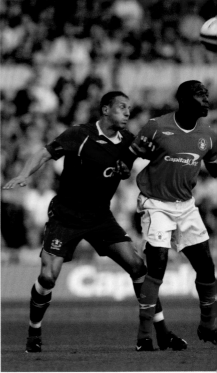

After so long with United, it felt strange to be up against friends like Rio Ferdinand.

A brief home-town swansong with Forest in 2008 turned out to be the last stop in my career.

Teddy Sheringham's failure to shake hands on my England debut in 1995 soured relations between us.

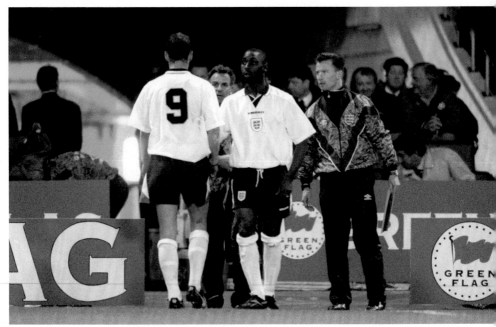

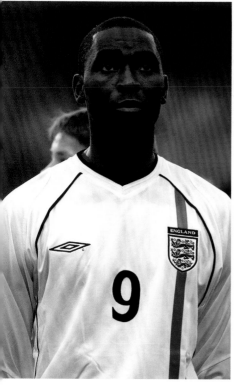

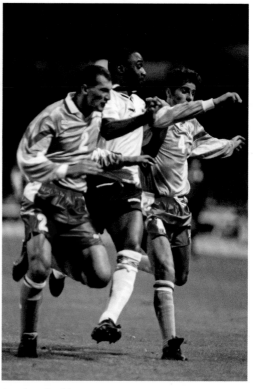

was always very proud to wear the Three Lions for England.

Sandwiched between two Uruguayan defenders at Wembley in my first international.

Reunited with my old Newcastle team-mate Peter Beardsley at an England get-together. Peter's football intelligence was off the charts.

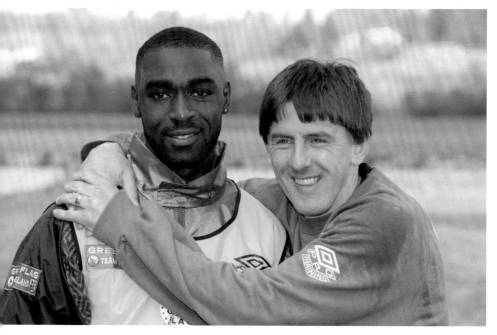

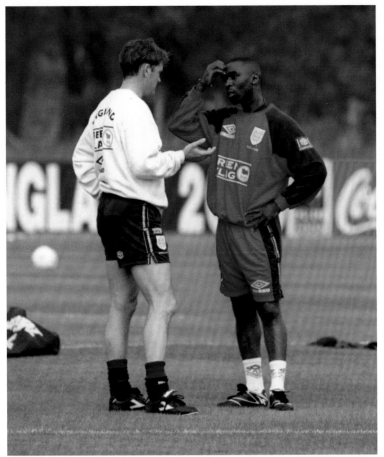

Left: Not the best communicator, Glenn Hoddle dropped me from the 1998 World Cup squad on dubious grounds.

Below: Back in the England fold in 2000 (here with Rio) and working with Kevin Keegan again.

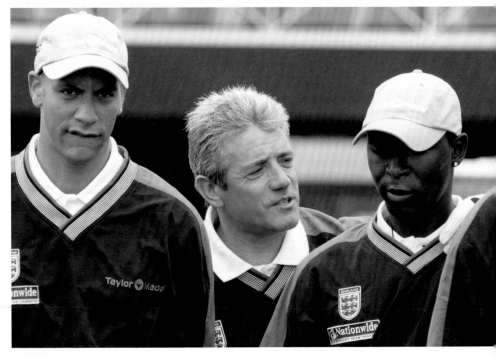

Right: Daddy cool! Holding my new son, Devante, in 1995 helped lift the gloom of losing the Premier League title to Blackburn.

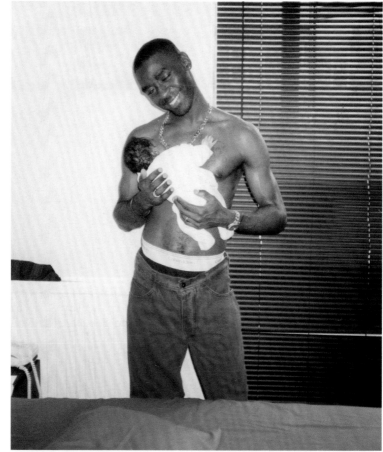

Below: Team Cole: Devante and my daughter, Faith, relax during a family holiday.

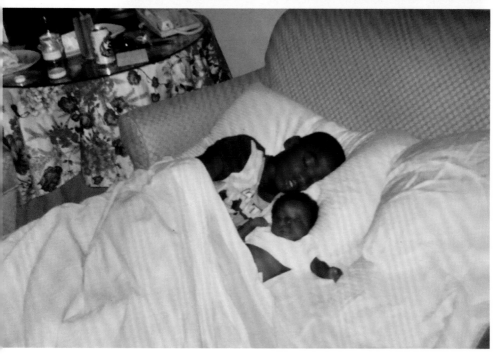

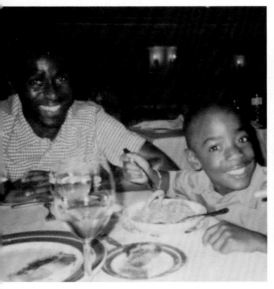

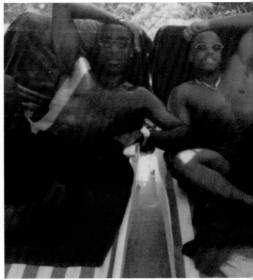

Enjoying a meal out with Devante. I am so proud of him.

Chilling in the sun with my nephew Kaymar. All my nephews have been incredibly supportive during my illness.

My hero! My consultant Mike Picton immediately knew just how ill I was and I'll always be grateful.

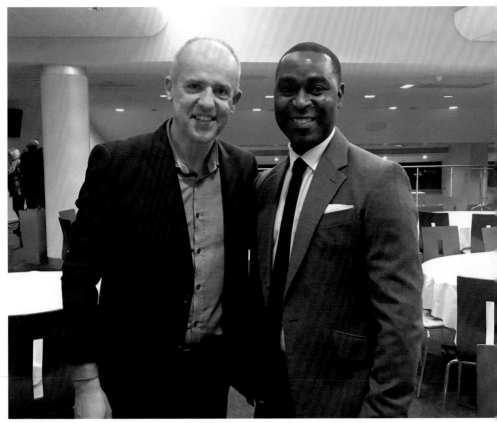

Right: My little angel, Faith, at my side after the 2017 kidney transplant. She has been an inspiration to me through my illness.

Below left: My grandparents were always a loving presence in my life.

Below right: Celebrating Father's Day with Devante and Faith. Everything I have ever done has been for my kids.

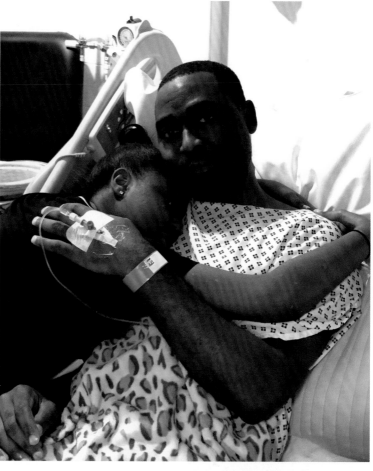

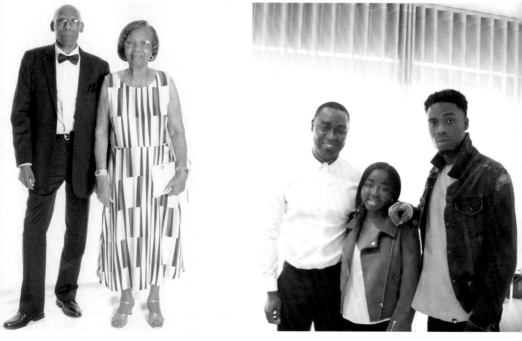

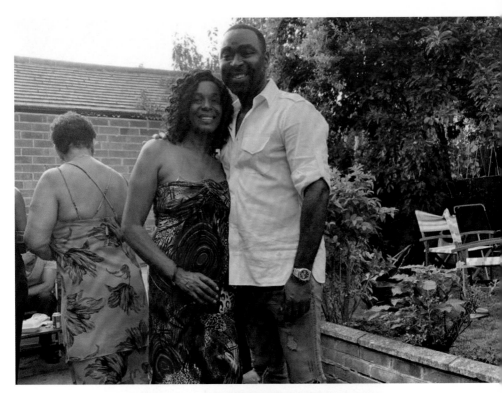

Above: My sister Jackie has always been like a second mum to me.

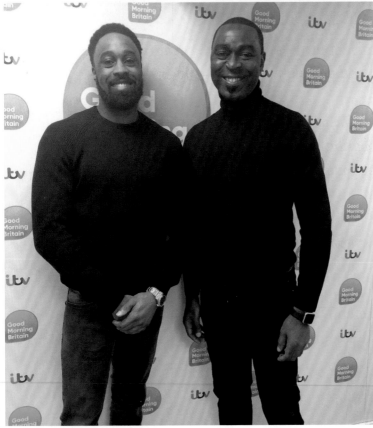

Left: Joined at the 2018 Good Morning Britain awards by my nephew Alexander. I will never be able to thank him enough for donating his kidney to me.

them up front, so much so that they had gone. I remember looking around late in the game and, yes, they had gone. You could see it in their eyes. A combination of absolute fatigue and bemusement. How had they been done by us? I got a late goal to win the match outright but we were already through. I am adamant about that. My goal only put a gloss on it, because the great Juventus had already been taken down.

In 2018, I was working for Manchester United in LA. We went for dinner at Alessandro Del Piero's restaurant, and he came over to have a good talk. 'I still can't believe what you did to us,' he said, the pain still etched around his eyes. 'I've never known how you, from that losing position, did such a job on us.' That's football. I feel the same about the Dortmund defeat in 1997. For all the wins, the defeats can still haunt us and perhaps always will.

A huge double blow that night was the suspension of Roy and Scholesy because of yellow cards. The dressing room was ablaze once again, 'We absolutely minced them!' was the constant shout, and these two strong men joined in, but a glance their way was enough to let them know how sorry you were.

The final stretch. We'd dropped a couple of points at Anfield at the beginning of May, despite being 2–0 up, but I scored at Leeds to salvage a big point (especially as Arsenal lost there) and we went into the last game knowing a win against Tottenham and we were champions. 'You're on the bench,' were not the words I wanted to hear. I was so hacked off but in the back of my mind I knew why.

That kiss-and-tell story had broken weeks before and I was struggling mentally. Life at home was tough, walking on glass every time I came through the door. Shirley was understandably unhappy and it was taking its toll. Mentally I was smashed and I think the gaffer could see that. Of course I argued with him, but deep down, I got it.

I was on at half-time. Les Ferdinand had put Spurs 1–0 up. I remember catching his eye from the bench as he ran back to his half, and he had this look in his eye. 'What the hell have I done?' He was my good mate but he was also probably aware that Tottenham fans wanted us to win the title, rather than Arsenal.

Becks scored a great equaliser just before half-time, but as we walked in the gaffer said, 'Teddy, you're coming off. Coley, get on.' No more than that, and so on I went and scored a goal that, four years after the game at West Ham that cost us the title, and despite winning two Premier Leagues since, finally brought me redemption.

Maybe it was the manner of the goal. One of my

best. Nev played a nice pass over the top and I spun in behind Sol Campbell, and I stretched to control the ball. In the corner of my eye I got an idea of Ian Walker's movement in goal. That's that picture I have talked about. When we were at Lilleshall together as kids, Ian had a reputation for having a little stroll. 'Walks' we used to call him. My mind was made up. He was coming off his line and so a lob and it was in.

We were 2–1 up and the Premier League was coming back. The celebrations were wild. Yorkey and I were rolling around the pitch like long-lost lovers. Not only did he know what Shirley and I were going through at home, but we had achieved something together, we'd become the most talked-about strike force in Europe and there was still so much more to look forward to.

Of the three trophies we won that season, the FA Cup final was the most straightforward. Getting to Wembley wasn't – the late win against Liverpool, beating Chelsea after a replay and that Arsenal epic. But the final, with all due respect to Newcastle, was a doddle.

I recently ran into Ruud Gullit, who was Newcastle's manager at the time, and he said, with a straight face, that he thought his team played very well and didn't deserve to lose. 'Are you joking, Ruud, we pummelled you,' was all I could say, because it was like a cat with a mouse. We lost Skip early to injury but Teddy came on and played very well, scoring one and setting up Scholesy for a second. We didn't have to get out of second gear, which was great considering the match we had on the following Wednesday, and we flew to Spain fresh and chilled.

We went to Barcelona on Concorde. We stayed in Sitges, a beautiful place, south-west of Barcelona. It was very chilled. There was no big fuss, just business as usual.

At Manchester United, you are very aware of what the competition means to the club, what the loss of those who died playing in it means. Munich is always with you when you play for the club, and being back in a final, we had to channel that emotion, use it, because it did seem like some things are meant to be. Now, I can say that with hindsight, but I do feel that special clubs can produce special moments.

It looked far from easy. We missed Roy and Scholesy but despite their absence I felt the team picked itself, even if it meant certain players playing out of position. Players like Giggsy and Becks, after all, were more than good enough to adapt. Giggsy could play anywhere. Left yes, but he played on the right on numerous occasions, he even played up front. Becks was of course so powerful on the right, but ask him, and he'd say he preferred centre midfield. Yes, losing two incredible players was going to hurt, but this was Manchester United, and there would be no excuses. Not rocket science. I was relaxed. I didn't usually get nervous. The lads used to say I could sleep on a washing line, but not that night. I was restless. I came down and the lads got talking and it seemed I wasn't alone. None of us had been involved in a game like this before. Everything else was familiar territory, the league and the FA Cup, but now we were on new ground, and that included the gaffer. Usually there was a bravado about the lads – no one would normally admit to any sort of nerves – and so it was strange to come down for breakfast and hear everyone being honest with each other and admitting to feeling the tension of the occasion.

What didn't change was that simple game plan. 'Go out there and enjoy it.'

It quickly became clear just how hard a game it was going to be. They scored a bad first-half goal and things were tight. Munich players have since told me that their game plan was stopping Yorkey and myself, which was kind of nice to hear, but at the time we huffed and puffed. It was a slog and they had the better chances.

They hit the bar and the post, but we had the gaffer's half-time words in our minds. He was so calm, simply saying don't get this close and lose, but for some reason we couldn't find a rhythm. I won't dress it up, we didn't play well, and when my number came up on eighty minutes, Ole got on and my final was over.

People ask me if I was disappointed, but I was only upset that we were losing. I wasn't going to sulk about coming off, and on the bench there was a continued belief. That trait that ran through the club of not giving up wasn't going to go away. I sat down, positive, knowing that the gaffer had made a move that he hoped would win us the Champions League.

A few had seen Lothar Matthäus smiling as if the job was over, but I didn't see it and anyway we had a very late corner. Come on! Becks swung it in, Peter Schmeichel was up and made a nuisance of himself, Giggsy scuffed it and I have to say Teddy half-scuffed it, but the ball was in the net and we were back in the game.

Steve McClaren had come in to replace Kiddo as assistant and I remember him trying to get some shape back, some calm. 'Four-four-two!' he was screaming, because we had no formation at that point, but we immediately won another corner and even the gaffer wasn't listening to him.

Becks again with the corner, Teddy's glancing header and Ole's toenail does the rest. Oh my God! We went nuts. I was by the corner flag before Ole. People who say I was upset coming off should ask how I got to the corner flag before him. I was ecstatic! It was bundle time. Bodies on top of bodies, screams of joy, total and utter happiness.

It was like being a kid when you used to jump on each other and make a pile. Moments that take you back to childhood. The flip side was our opponents. Sammy Kuffour, Munich's brilliant centre-back and a player I had the utmost respect for, was lying on the ground, smashing his fist down on the turf, like a toddler denied his favourite ice-cream. That's the game. These moments make kids of us all and while we bundled on top of each other, Sammy was left in despair.

For us, everything went out of the window. Pierluigi Collina, the ref, tried to get us all off, but it was going to take a minute and there wasn't any time left to play. We were European Champions. Raw passion. Raw emotion. I ran to the fans, a group of supporters who always had my back. I don't know why, but I must have done something right. Early on in my time at the club, a team-mate said, 'Do you know how lucky you are? They have a song about you,' and from there, through hard times and now the best of times, I went to them and together we celebrated.

Twenty years later, that reunion at Old Trafford and it was so nice to see everyone's faces, to have the same old laughs and jokes, and to be stupid again. Life as you grow older can be hard, but when you sit with a group of lads like the Treble-winning squad at Manchester United, worries and stresses just drop away. We were back at Old Trafford, but we were also in Turin, we were at Villa Park, we were at the Nou Camp. Whatever happens and however much time passes, I guess we always will be.

11

BLAME IT ON RIO

Copacabana beach curves into the distance. The blue Atlantic laps up to its white sand, while Sugar Loaf Mountain gives a thumbs-up in the distance by way of approval. Christ the Redeemer overlooks the scene, his arms spread as if not quite believing the sheer beauty of his surroundings. We're high above Rio de Janeiro. We have a day off. Told to relax by the gaffer, the lads are recharging their batteries by the hotel pool, but four of us have made a break for it.

'Let's go paragliding.'

I can't remember who said it, but Roy Keane, Nicky Butt, Ryan Giggs and I are climbing a hill, ready to make the leap over the beauty of Rio.

'Hold on, what's the date?' I ask.

'It's Friday,' says Giggsy.

'Not the day, the date.'

'Oh, it's the thirteenth.'

Now, I'm not the most superstitious man around, but I'm getting out of there. There is no way I am jumping off a mountain and floating on the wind on Friday the thirteenth. 'See you later.' I get myself back down to the safety of sea level and head back to the hotel.

The thing to know here is, activities like paragliding are frowned upon at football clubs like Manchester United, even if strapped to instructors as they are going to be. Managers and contracts tend to steer their multi-million-pound assets away from such extreme sports.

I sit back down by the pool and it's not long before you can hear shouts coming from high above. 'Oi, ****heads!' We all look around before looking up. 'Down there, you ****heads!' High above the hotel, three bird-like figures, hovering, shouting their abuse. 'What a bunch of ****heads.'

As the lads look confused, I'm trying not to laugh. The gaffer sits up from his sun lounger and says, 'Who the hell are those idiots?'

I shake my head, trying to suppress even a smile. 'Must be a few tourists who don't like United, boss,' I say.

'Idiots.'

I'm trying so hard not to laugh but force myself to keep quiet because if the gaffer finds out it's three of his players up there, he will go ballistic.

Eventually the flying three returned. I got some stick for not taking the leap with them, but at least I never named names. I love looking back on my time in football and smiling at little stories such as this one. Not only was I playing for one of the biggest clubs in world football, not only was I playing in the best competitions and seeing the world, but I was making the best friends and sharing memories that today still make me laugh. Life has thrown stuff at me since I retired, but to be able to look back and think of those three multiple Premier League-winners shouting abuse from the Rio skies seems to brighten the greyest of days.

One day it ends. Everyone has to leave Manchester United and my day would come, but after the highs of the Treble season, the big challenge was getting motivated to do it all again. With our gaffer that was never going to be too hard. It was a message he drummed into us. Last season was last season, never look back, defending trophies is motivation in itself.

For me personally, my summer helped to ground me. Just a week after the immense highs of Barcelona and the homecoming to a sea of red in Manchester, I took myself to Africa. I had started the 'Andy Cole Foundation' and travelled to Zimbabwe to see the work we were doing out there.

The charity was set up to help children and when I saw how they lived their lives day to day but still kept smiling and moving forward, not only was I immediately grounded but everything was quickly put in perspective.

Any thoughts about how great I was and how amazing my recent achievements had been disappeared the second I got a closer look at the poverty that the people and the children there were (and still are) subject to.

Homelessness, despair, hunger – all met with dignity and even humour. The children smiling, excited to see you, not an ounce of self-pity. So many kids sleeping rough, just children. There was no food, and any money they had was worthless. I arrived thinking I was some sort of hero. I left knowing who the real heroes were.

There was this myth going around that AIDS (a massive problem out there) could be cured by sleeping with a young virgin. Children were suffering and it affected me. I wanted to help and in a small way we did, but I returned home re-evaluating my life.

Today, I still think of those children in Zimbabwe. In the western world, we all live in a bubble. Our own little worlds. My own kids do, and it's so easy to become numb to any other problems. Today people have their phones, their iPads, Netflix. That summer, in 1999, I had my Premier League medal, my FA Cup medal, my Champions League medal, but I was brought back to earth with a bump, coming face to face with the reality of a bigger, harder world. I never let my kids forget about it.

That experience actually helped me come back to football. I had seen there was more to life than training and playing and the television and the newspapers. I was still hungry to achieve things in the game, but I was definitely aware of a bigger picture and made decisions to expand my boundaries.

People ask what you can achieve after a Treble. That summer I had a go at trying to break the top forty. My agent knew someone in the music industry, and knowing my love of hip hop, it was put to me: 'Fancy making a record?'

In years gone by, I might have shied away from the idea. Maybe it was the Treble success, more likely it was my trip to Africa, but why not? Why not step out of my comfort zone? It's OK to have a bit of fun.

And it was a lot of fun. From a young age, I have been surrounded by music. From old reggae to my own love of rap music, it has always been a big part of my life. Music cheers the soul, and despite knowing the stick I would take from the lads, I dived into it, making a video and having a ball.

The song didn't do that well, but I'm proud if it. I took a lot of banter for that one. It would be playing when I walked into a dressing room, it would come on in the team bus. Listen, I brought up the big issues, drugs, crime, all of it. In the video I was in the passenger seat of a car. I'm not sure why I wasn't driving while I rapped. Maybe they thought I couldn't multi-task! Even today, people will bring it up. In fact, Devante

– now he is a footballer, and thanks largely to YouTube – gets stick too, so I think he's pretty happy that I never went for the follow-up record.

I took all the banter that came my way after that record on the chin. The public's perception of me might be this introspective, serious type, but my mates will tell you, mates I have been going on holiday with for over twenty years, that I am happiest when on a night out, getting and giving out stick. Trust me, my little stint in show business armed my mates for quite a few years . . . and still rears its head today. No regrets, though. I think it's a tune!

Living in and around Manchester in the late 1990s was big for any music lover. Britpop was never really my thing, but we did get to see the members of Stone Roses at times as they were big reds. Noel and Liam Gallagher were less likely to be seen at Old Trafford, but it was an exciting time and the city I called home for twenty-five years was at its vibrant best. The people there are so nice and so welcoming, and at the time they could boast to be living in the cultural heartland of Cool Britannia.

Pre-season after the Treble was far from an oasis. The gaffer was even more focused, more hungry for success, and if anything it was even more intense. Alongside the manager now was Steve McClaren. We all liked Steve. He was young, not much older than us, had fresh ideas, he was vibrant, and settled in quickly.

Not that I didn't keep him on his toes. As I did with most coaches, I would test Steve. I remember the gaffer wanted to see me once and sent Steve to bring me to his office. I knew what was happening, the gaffer was going to tell me I wasn't playing at the weekend, and I wasn't in the mood. 'I'm not coming,' I said.

'What?'

'I'm not coming.'

Steve's face was a picture. I saw him recently and he said, 'You were a nightmare, Coley.' Just keeping you on your toes, Steve.

He would go on to be a good manager in his own right, but I remember being on a pre-season tour without the gaffer when Steve was 'in charge'. We were allowed one night out and ended up in the hotel club, having a few beers. Steve came over and looked at his watch.

'Right, lads, it's quarter to midnight. Finish your drinks and get to your rooms.'

A bit later, when our bottles of beer had been refilled, he came over again.

'Right, lads, it's quarter past twelve, time for bed.'

We all nodded, but at half past he was back, ushering us all out. Every one of us, every single one, went upstairs – and came straight back down. Steve was left finishing his beer, watching us all walk back in, one by one. He gave up on us and we finished at around 5 a.m.

Let me tell you, training the next morning was the funniest sight. A load of supposedly highly tuned athletes struggling to even move. At one point, Yorkey went to the floor to do up his laces and just lay down and fell asleep. We were all squirting water at him, but nothing. He was out. We were in hysterics. Steve had no choice but to cancel the session. It was no good, we were mullered.

The pre-season after the Treble was spent in Australia. Today such trips are the norm, but back then they were quite rare and it proved that Manchester United wanted to capitalise on its success and take the 'brand' global.

I had never been Down Under before and loved being there. The bonding between the lads was great, but the trip turned sour for me when an opponent suffered a nasty injury.

It was our second game and we were playing the national team. I went for a tackle with a rising star of the Australian game, a young lad called Simon Colosimo, but caught him on his knee and he did his cruciate. Out of the game for over a year.

The media out there suggested I had done it on

purpose. The British press picked up on it and suddenly I was this thuggish player who went out to deliberately hurt the kid. It was a bad tackle, I accept that, but I was going for the ball and I missed. That was all. I mistimed it and caught the lad's knee. Unfortunately it happens, and to suggest I had been malicious was plain wrong.

Then there was the suggestion that I hadn't apologised. I was very sorry that he had got injured, but I had nothing to say sorry for. It's football. We were challenging for the ball and he got hurt. Anyone who knows me knows that I would never seek to hurt someone. I'll look after myself, but that sort of behaviour is simply not my bag. But there it was, things were being written about me without any justification.

In the build-up to the season, lots had also been written about who would replace Peter Schmeichel in the Manchester United goal. Whoever did was always going to find it tough, but that season we had two keepers who, for different reasons, would struggle to narrow the angles set by one of the true greats.

First of all there was Mark Bosnich. Just thinking about Boso makes me laugh. He was a great lad but he arrived at the club a little overweight and was told by the gaffer to lose it. Many people see Boso as this party boy, but let me tell you, he worked his arse off in training to get fit. He'd just got married, was very professional and actually Boso was a great keeper.

A brilliant shot-stopper, he struggled a bit with his feet. Back then, keepers weren't being asked to start attacks the way they are today, but Boso couldn't kick the ball any distance. He just couldn't get through it. The ball used to spin back like a golf shot and the lads would laugh, saying that he must be wearing Sinbad's shoes.

He was funny. We were once playing Leeds. Boso hadn't been there long and the gaffer was giving a pre-match talk over breakfast. He was just about to get started when Boso stood up and said, 'Sorry, boss, I'm just going to get some eggs.' He was met with silence and terror. We all looked at the gaffer, but I think he was too shocked to even give out a bollocking.

As well as Boso, we had Massimo Taibi. Max was such a lovely guy. We all got on with him, but the Italian struggled and some high-profile mistakes took their toll. It's hard to see guys you genuinely like go through that. He made a mistake against Southampton that was shown again and again. He was a great pro and he worked so hard, but at a club like Manchester United the way you start is so vital. I always feel for keepers, because we all make mistakes but theirs, as we all know, lead to goals, and goals lead to scrutiny. Max had no chance after his mistakes.

The gaffer had also added the French defender Mikaël Silvestre and South African midfielder Quinton Fortune to the squad. Fortune was so popular. I'm not exaggerating when I say he is one of the nicest people I have ever met. A great footballer, strong and skilful, he was a great addition to the squad, but when you are at a club where Roy Keane and Paul Scholes play in your position, game time is always going to be hard to come by.

The gaffer, though, was a genius at keeping a squad happy. It's a bit like spinning plates, as everyone wants to play, but he had a knack of making everybody feel part of the season. Reassuring footballers and keeping them able to jump out of bed of a morning, eager to come in and contribute, is not easy, but the gaffer always managed to do just that and then, often at vital moments in a season, a player would pop up and win an awkward victory.

For me, the season started well. At the end of August, Newcastle came to Old Trafford. We beat them 5–1 and I got four goals. It was just one of those days. The weather was great, the team were great and everything I hit went in. I'm not sure about 'the zone', but there are days when it all goes for you and we just kept opening them up.

I have quite a few match balls from hat-tricks scored, but don't ask me where they are. Someone's loft, I guess. I'll find them all some day and I'm sure that that one would be signed by the lads, saying things like 'You should have scored five.' My medals are in safety-deposit boxes now, but things like match balls and shirts might be harder to locate.

The season started well enough for the team, too. A 5–0 drubbing at Chelsea was a strange one, but there was no hangover from that or the Treble season as we steamed into Christmas, picking up win after win. By now, though, we knew that our January would be different from normal as the club had accepted FIFA's invitation to play in the Club World Championship in Brazil. It was an exciting thought, but the fact that it meant we would not be around to defend the FA Cup caused a bit of a stir.

The gaffer was under attack from those who felt the club had disrespected the FA Cup, but I think he had his hands tied – under pressure from the FA to take part and possibly help a future World Cup bid – and while it was suggested that we could play a youth team in the early rounds, there was no way the gaffer would go for that.

As players, we were just told we were going, and so the focus was on heading out there wanting to win it. We started off playing Necaxa of Mexico at the famous Maracanã. It was hot. Mad hot. At home or in Europe,

I always wore long sleeves whatever the weather, but this was different. Over 100 degrees, and the tops we had brought with us were the usual thick ones. Our kit man, Albert Morgan, looked on in shock as we all took scissors to the sleeves. 'Sorry, Bert, but you're taking the mickey with these tops.'

We got out on the pitch and I remember lining up for the anthems and taking in my surroundings. The Maracanã. It was in a bit of a state back then, but I couldn't stop thinking of the players who had gone before us. Pelé, Zico, Sócrates. I stood there, looked around and thought about where I'd come from.

'Maybe I've half cracked this,' I said to myself. 'I have worked hard and football has taken me to the most special of places, and here I am, about to play at the Maracanã. Not bad at all.'

The football didn't go as well as the daydreaming. We drew that game against the Mexicans and then faced the Brazilian team, Vasco da Gama. I was on the bench that night but was almost brought off my seat when their striker, Edmundo, scored the naughtiest goal I have ever seen. We were already two goals down, thanks to a Romário brace, but when the ball was knocked into their striker, he was marked by Silvestre. He stabbed the ball into the ground, let the spin move it around his marker, turned with it, and slipped it past Bosnich in our goal. Ridiculous!

I think I might even have clapped. Think of Dennis Bergkamp against Newcastle for Arsenal in 2002. I rate Dennis, and what a goal his was, but this was even better in its execution. Poor Mikaël. He was turned inside out and it was a reminder of where we were, a place where even on the beach across from our hotel, there were kids and girls and guys showing us skills that made our toes curl.

We won our last game but had been eliminated from the competition. The gaffer was upset – everything we played he wanted to win – but he looked ahead at the season and told us to spend the rest of the short time left there to relax. Get rested and be ready to get straight back into the swing of things at home. And apart from those men in their flying machines, that's just what we did.

In the end, the trip to Rio wasn't the best PR exercise, we didn't do well on the pitch, Martin Edwards was photographed dancing with a Brazilian lady who looked like she might have been paid to be danced with ('Go on, the Chairman!') and we returned home to loads of headlines about our disrespect for the world's oldest cup competition.

There was a new attitude in English football: 'Anyone But United'. We'd become public enemies, but as players you don't care. You don't care about other teams when they're doing well, because it's out of your control, and you certainly don't care what people think of you when you're doing well, because usually it's just petty. It's up to them to catch you.

The *Daily Mirror* started a campaign to save the FA Cup. The editor at the time was Piers Morgan, an Arsenal fan with an Arsenal agenda. He hasn't changed, has he? As a Manchester United player you became used to snide comments, but that's all they were. If anything, they helped the gaffer, who thrived on creating a siege mentality.

While we had been away in Brazil, no one had taken advantage of our absence. Like an F1 driver taking a pitstop only to come back out on the track still in the lead, we were under no pressure. We even managed to draw our first two league games back, the second one against Arsenal, but went top after the following fixture and stayed there, winning ninety-one points, to take the league by eighteen points.

The defence of the Champions League proved less successful. Real Madrid knocked us out at the quarter-final stage and once again we were left with regrets. We should have won at the Bernabéu – I had a great chance to score but got too much on a header – but still, we came home with a goalless draw. Confidence turned to dismay when we were beaten at home by the best team in the competition, thanks largely to a bit of skill from Fernando Redondo. Not quite as good as Edmundo's a few weeks earlier, but still so dirty and right up there with the best I've seen. Poor Henning Berg had done everything right, pushing the midfielder wide, but a back-heel around our defender and he was in to square for the brilliant Raúl to do the rest.

Steve McManaman was playing for Madrid that night, and would win his second Champions League later that season. Many people have asked if I fancied moving abroad and I have to say I didn't. There was a moment when Juventus were said to be interested, but it didn't become anything more than paper talk and, if I'm honest, when I was at my peak at Old Trafford, the Premier League was so exciting, every game so big a challenge, my team so good, that there was nowhere else I wanted to be.

Football, though, cares little for what we want, and it wasn't long before it looked very much like I'd have to move on. The summer of 2000, and the gaffer's interest in the Dutch striker Ruud van Nistelrooy was more than mere newspaper talk. He was coming, and for a lot of money. The club were going to cash in on me to help finance their £19 million signing and it was time to find a new home. It was going to be Chelsea.

Gianluca Vialli was the manager at Stamford Bridge and he wanted me to play up front with Jimmy Floyd Hasselbaink. My agent brokered a deal with the chief executive, Colin Hutchinson, and the move was very nearly done. The money was good, Manchester United were getting the fee they wanted, I even went online to look at houses down there. It was just a case of signing the contract and then, bang, Ruud's knee went in training at PSV in Holland and everything changed.

Football, like life, is strange. It's like that movie, *Sliding Doors*. Things can change in a flash. As I talked to Chelsea and thought about my new future, I wasn't exactly doing cartwheels. I didn't want to leave United, I loved the club, it was my club, and so, if I'm brutally honest, I was the only winner when Ruud's knee injury proved too serious for him to sign. Another player's misfortune can be to your benefit, and after being days away from leaving, I was signing a new contract at Old Trafford and looking forward to defending the title in red once again. From packing my kit bag to being straight back in and motivated.

The gaffer that summer was all about winning a third consecutive Premier League title. A hat-trick of championships is rare, achieved by only a few clubs, and as ever we set out to make history. Like the previous season, with our rivals either in transition or, frankly, not good enough, we won it by ten points.

I didn't play as many games as I would have liked in 2000–01 but still managed to get thirteen goals in all competitions and enjoyed more goalscoring feats in the Champions League. My hat-trick at home to Anderlecht in the group stages stands out and I was desperate to experience another Champions League final.

Unfortunately, we came up against Bayern Munich in the quarter-final, a team as desperate as us but also out for revenge. We were beaten home and away and once again it was a matter of close but no cigar. So often we were beaten by the team who went on to win the Champions League, but that was no consolation.

Losing in the quarter- or semi-finals is a killer. Giggsy used to say you can smell the hot dogs, and he was so right. We were always good enough, and I look back with massive regret that we didn't win the Champions League two or three times while I was there.

The 2001–02 season started with the departure of a big figure. Jaap Stam had been a huge part of our recent success. One of the best centre-backs I ever saw, the big man left suddenly in the first week of the season. We had played Fulham at home and Jaap had been up against Louis Saha. Now, Louis was a brilliant footballer and he was lightning. Jaap, no slouch himself, had had surgery on his Achilles and was trying to get back to speed. He had a good few yards on Louis, but the French striker put his burners on and Jaap looked like the tortoise chasing the hare.

The next week he was gone. That's harsh, we all thought. A lot was made about a book Jaap had published, but the gaffer simply thought that, taking into account the big money being offered by Lazio and the Dutchman's age (he was thirty), it was wise to sell. I know the gaffer later regretted the decision, because he was still one of the best around, but even the greats make mistakes.

It was a time when Sir Alex was having to think more about players and what they did away from football. Becks by now was a national celebrity, married to a pop star and constantly on the front pages of magazines and papers. The gaffer was no fan of all that, but the money in the game was getting huge and he would have to get used to it.

My mate Yorkey was no stranger to a glossy magazine. Whereas I saw playing for Manchester United as the job I loved, Dwight continued to enjoy the benefits that come with it. I remember him coming to me and saying he was going out with the model Jordan, or Katie Price. He asked what I thought, and of course it was simply a case of whatever makes you happy.

Katie used to come to games and the papers were all over her relationship with Victoria Beckham, saying there was a problem, but for me she was my mate's girlfriend and seemed nice. I might have been different from Yorkey, but you just want your mates to be happy. Dwight kept it all in check, though. The minute you see yourself as a celebrity rather than a footballer, you are in trouble and, for all the red carpets, he knew that.

I knew that season was going to be tricky. Scrap that, not tricky, it was going to be a challenge. Ruud van Nistelrooy was fit and on his way and the gaffer's squad was starting to take a new shape. Laurent Blanc came in to replace Jaap and showed his sheer class immediately. He was never quick, but what a footballer. Juan Sebastián Verón came in too and, wow, some talent.

The things the Argentine did in training. He would control the ball with the sole of his boot and nutmeg us all for fun. 'The Little Witch', they used to call him, and he would put spells on us most days. He was also one of the nicest men I have ever met. One day I asked if he could pick me up a Rolex Daytona watch from Argentina, as they were limited and unavailable in the UK. He brought one back and when I asked to arrange paying him, he said, 'No, this is for your birthday, my friend.'

He was one of the lads, and when it came to the gaffer's plans, he was one of the forwards. In Europe, especially, the gaffer was looking to change things. He wanted Ruud up top on his own, with Seb in behind him. Ruud was fine with that. I liked him a lot, but he preferred going alone. '*I can do this stuff myself!*'

A lone striker was becoming all the rage across the continent and the gaffer had bought the talent to implement that, but it was going to make my life awkward. I wanted to play, I particularly wanted to play in the Champions League, a competition I loved, and while I was ready to fight my way back into his plans, I knew that this time the gaffer was going to be a hard nut to crack.

As the season got going, I was on at him regularly. 'Play me' became my motto. We had a meeting and I explained that I wanted to play football. I wasn't a good substitute. My dad and grandad had always told me to work hard and that nothing comes for free. You have to work to get by, and sitting in a tracksuit didn't feel like working to me.

Too many players back then, at clubs everywhere, were signing three- or four-year contracts and happily sitting games out. Come on. Where's your ambition? That wasn't for me, and I think, deep down, the gaffer knew that. Another meeting. 'I'm nicking a living,' I told him. He would reassure me, saying I would get my fill, but I wasn't satisfied.

I would go and see him two or three times a week.

'Play me!' He would laugh at my impatience, but he respected my desire to play. It became a ritual. 'Play me!' Some days he could hear me coming towards his office and I'd hear, 'Get lost, Coley, I'm not in the mood today.'

We would actually laugh about it, but my mind was constantly ticking. The 2002 World Cup was on the horizon. Sven-Göran Eriksson had told me I was in his plans, but I knew I needed to be playing regularly and scoring goals. In January of that year, exactly seven years after joining from Newcastle, I made the decision. I was going to leave.

The gaffer tried to make me change my mind. I had two years left on my contract, but he knew me. We'd worked so well together in that seven years, but now I had an itch. Time to go. It's never easy to walk away from a club like Manchester United. I had walked in a promising striker under pressure, but I had been coached, supported, loved by the fans, and ultimately we were all successful.

I had more football to play elsewhere, life had more challenges to throw at me, but the club never leaves you. Today I can bowl into the stadium or the training ground and I am treated as one of the players. We may be talking about a global super-club, but it's that feeling of family that outshines the razzmatazz. Once you're in, you're always in. I was looking for new adventures, but I would never forget my past.

12

BREAK THE ICE

Graeme Souness could sell ice to the Eskimos. A charmer, a smooth operator, a manager able to sell me a dream. One of the greats as a player and as smooth with his mouth as he once was with his feet. I left Manchester United still wanting to do so much in the game, and it was Graeme who convinced me I could do all that with him, but in time things got so bad between us, so fractious, that my position at the club became completely untenable. I had to leave. If I hadn't, something bad would have happened. I would have been sacked. Or arrested.

When I decided to leave Manchester United, not an easy decision for any footballer, I was after a new home, somewhere I wouldn't merely wind down, but a place to retire while still striving to learn; a place to get better, help younger players improve; somewhere to achieve as much as I could in the short time my career had left.

I have talked about a picture I would get in my head when I was in on goal. I also had pictures about my career. I had been lucky enough to achieve so much already but I was hungry for more, and when I had my first meeting with Graeme, the things he told me fitted perfectly with everything I wanted from the rest of my career.

Graeme and I had met at his apartment. We spoke for a bit and I left thinking, 'Why not?' I was so impressed by him. He had said all the right things. He talked about what we could both achieve. He had a vision of where the club might go and he emphasised the importance of my role in that vision. He told me that I had loads of goals left in me, that I would play games and that I could be a massive help to the young, talented players at the club.

My own personal desire to play in that summer's World Cup was immediate, but I liked how long-term Graeme's own ambitions were. The side were actually struggling when we met, but he told me they just lacked a bit of class, and that I was that class. Everything seemed right, including the location.

My main focus was my kids, and with Devante still at a primary school we very much liked, we wanted to stay in the north-west. It all just seemed perfect, and in many ways it was. Blackburn Rovers was the love-liest of clubs. The nicest staff worked there, the fans were great, all good Lancashire people. The squad was exceptional, so much so you wondered how the hell they were doing so badly. Surely that couldn't last. It all felt very right when I walked into my new place of work.

Seeing Old Trafford getting smaller in the rear-view mirror of your career is hard. You can never forget the sound of the Stretford End roaring a goal you've scored, or singing your name; you can never stop thinking about European nights at Old Trafford, those floodlights beaming down on us, our wingers bombing forward as we chase a late goal, the whole stadium willing us on with so much passion, you wondered if the roof would lift off.

You can't put all that to one side, and neither did I want to, but I wasn't leaving with an ounce of self-pity. I am not one to look backwards. I prefer to keep moving forward, and that's what I did, all the way up the short section of the M61 to Ewood Park.

What I immediately liked about Blackburn as a club was how friendly it was. It reminded me of Old Trafford. That might sound odd, considering the difference in sizes, but the people, being practically neighbours, were so similar and so welcoming.

The big difference is the level of expectation. Blackburn might have won the Premier League seven years earlier, but they had since been relegated and promoted, and while Graeme was clearly ambitious to achieve things, the general feel from the club and the fans was a world away from Manchester United.

That wasn't a problem. You have to put pressure on yourself. I always had and I wasn't going to stop there. I actually relished the challenge. I'd bounce out of bed: we had a cup to win. One of my first games was at Sheffield Wednesday in the League Cup semi-final. I scored and we would make it to the final. A final. No worries about still wanting to achieve things, then. Keep moving forward.

With my powers of self-motivation I must have been an easy player for Graeme to manage – at first. He actually used to make me laugh, but not intentionally. First of all, there was the way he joined in all the sessions. Aged fifty-plus but still keen to show us all how good he was. It became a problem later, but for now I would have a giggle as he chased us around the training pitches.

Don't get me wrong, Graeme Souness was some footballer. You could have nothing but respect for what he did in the game. The captain he became, the competitor he was and the trophies he won. The thing is, he liked to tell us all about them.

'Coley, how many European Cups have you won?'

'One, boss.'

'Oh, is that all? I think it was my third when we won in Rome, against Roma.'

It was funny. The players would smile, but it could get a bit cringe-making at times. Maybe he wanted to be one of the lads, but I didn't take him too seriously, and to be honest, his past was of no interest when things were going so badly for Blackburn. Before I arrived, the team had lost five out of six games. I managed to score on my Ewood Park debut in a 4–1 win against Charlton, but we then lost the next four league games and, no matter what we had all achieved in our pasts, our present saw us bang in trouble.

I did not want a relegation on my CV and, looking around the dressing room, you had to wonder why we were looking up at most of the other teams: Brad Friedel in goal, great pros like Henning Berg, Stig Inge Bjornebye, Craig Short, Mark Hughes, Tugay. Promising youngsters like Matt Jansen, David Dunn and Damien Duff.

'Too good to go down' was the dreaded phrase being thrown about, but we as a group knew there was hard work to be done. That's when I started to get a bit concerned. It dawned on me that the training at Rovers just wasn't good enough.

Graeme had his old mate Phil Boersma as his coach and Phil would take the training, including the fitness stuff. The warm-ups were an absolute joke. It was as if we, the squad, professional footballers, were warming him up.

I got the impression that Phil might have liked the odd beer or glass of wine at night. He'd come in, get his tracksuit on and he'd run us, at whatever pace he chose, around the whole perimeter of the training ground. We'd all be looking baffled at each other, but it happened every morning and you have to wonder if it was so he could sweat out the couple of drinks he'd had the night before.

I was saying to myself, I know I am not the best trainer in the world, but this is ridiculous. He should be warming us up, not the other way around. He's getting a good sweat on, but we certainly weren't getting much out of it.

And then there were the sessions. Small-sided games. Over and over again. After a few weeks, I realised it wasn't going to change. It was so monotonous, lacking intensity, and the team were suffering. It wasn't long before I voiced my opinion.

Graeme and Phil would always say it was what they did at Liverpool and I respected that. I respected what Liverpool achieved, of course I did, but the reason they could hone their game with small-sided games was because they had the best players in Europe. This Blackburn group needed coaching. We were good players, but as a group we needed preparing for the weekend – put on a session, work on aspects of the team that needed it. Instead, the management focused on things individuals couldn't do, but only as a way of showing that individual up. 'How come you can't do that?' was the shout. I got frustrated. Phil would say, 'You can't make chicken salad out of chicken shit,' a line I found disrespectful. It was a cop-out. You're the coach, coach the bloody team. Make us better!

I was becoming visibly despondent. Ironic, really, when I had spent the majority of my career training as casually as I could, always getting exactly what I wanted from it, but this was just wrong. The team needed guidance. I realised I had been spoilt at Manchester United, where training was always bang on, but I hadn't come here to knock off. Sign a three-year contract, put the slippers on, light a cigar – that's not me, but this training, the same every day, it wasn't on.

It made me feel sluggish, my mood darkened and I would say my bit. Maybe they started to see me as a troublemaker, but what else could I do? Mark Hughes saw it was worrying me and told me not to let it rile me. Easier said than done. I wasn't enjoying going into training because I wasn't getting what I wanted from it.

What I did like was my team-mates. A great bunch of lads, and a fine group of footballers. A lot of the players had been Championship players, wanting to get to the next level. You could see they wanted more. I'm sure if you asked anyone there, young players such as Dunny or Duff, who moved on to other clubs, they would tell you that the training at Rovers wasn't enough.

Sorry for mentioning Manchester United again, but it was there that my standards were set. I understand not everyone can reach Sir Alex Ferguson's levels, but it was simple really. Keep the players on their toes, take them to one side now and then, tell them they are lacking in something and then work on it with them.

Make every day different. Variety is the spice of life and footballers need stimulating. Phil's dreaded warm-up and constant small-sided games? No, thanks. Not happening. I was almost in my mid-thirties, a footballing OAP according to most, but I was still keen to learn and get a buzz from the everyday, and I was just as keen to see young footballers get better and maybe help them a bit along the way.

You want to pull players up to your level. That's not me being flash, that is what most senior pros want to do. You want to pass on knowledge, make young players better, just as the likes of Peter Beardsley had done with me when I was starting out.

There was a lot of promising talent at Blackburn. But they needed coaching, guidance. Matty Jansen was one.

A lot of potential. A magic left foot and bundles of skill. What he needed help with was his decision-making. He could hog the ball. Wouldn't get his head up. He'd beat a couple, but he'd want to make that a few, and if he did give it to you, it was because there was nothing more he felt he could do with it. By then, space had been denied, the chance gone. He could have been coached, because with the ability to truly get his head up and see pictures in front of him, Matty could have played at the highest level. He was also very unlucky with a nasty head injury when he was hit by a car in Rome whilst riding a scooter. I liked him a lot.

Dunny was the same. Loads of ability. Good passer, loved Gazza and wanted to beat men like him, but again he needed help with his decision-making. Damien Duff was one who did have it all. All he lacked, in fact, was a bit of self-belief, but that came, and you could see from his time at Chelsea that this was a player who met the highest standards. Duffer actually turned down Manchester United for Chelsea, but I wasn't at all surprised by how well he did there. He had this effortless skill. He would get it rolled into him, and he'd roll it off his left foot and turn inside, so natural the full-back would think he couldn't get near him. He'd scoot inside, drop his shoulder, go back outside. It was a joy to watch, and a pleasure to play with.

As well as the youngsters there, we had plenty of solid quality and experience. Big Craig Short at the back. It makes me laugh to think that he and I had a bit of a run-in one day in training – he's massive! But we're good friends now. Martin Taylor was a good defender, 6 ft 4 in but he'd get beaten in the air by forwards who were 5 ft 10 in. If he'd had Shorty's aggression, he'd have been some player. Garry Flitcroft, a great lad and a great pro. Keith Gillespie was there. Keith had his demons by now, but you could never accuse him of giving anything less than everything on a match day.

Then there was Tugay. I called him the Mad Turk. What a funny guy. I got on with him very well. He smoked like a chimney, but he was some footballer. Not much running, but great ability. He could do these no-look passes, always finding my runs. An exquisite footballer.

Yes, the ability was there. Results would follow in time but during those early defeats, it was hard to get used to losing games. Not just losing games, but going into games not solely focused on winning. You have to adapt, but there were niggling worries. Do all of my team-mates really fancy it today, especially when we played the better teams?

*

As I looked around the dressing room at Cardiff's Millennium Stadium, I had no such fears. You can never doubt Graeme's competitive streak, and we were a well-motivated team that Sunday for the League Cup final against Tottenham in February 2002.

I was desperate to win the League Cup. That will sound funny to some, the snobs who continue to say, 'It's only the League Cup.' Try telling Pep Guardiola that, who seems more than happy to win it. Players and managers want to win things, and having won everything else at Manchester United, I was hungry to complete the set.

A few papers made a thing about me facing Glenn Hoddle at Tottenham, and Teddy Sheringham too, but neither even crossed my mind. This was about Blackburn. Not many gave us a chance. Tottenham had a good side and we were in the bottom three of the Premier League, but we embraced the occasion, thrived on the atmosphere – the roof was on and the noise was loud – and we played well.

Matt Jansen put us one up, but Spurs, as expected, came at us hard and got an equaliser. We never stopped competing, though. Dunny was keeping possession well, Sparky was in midfield and, even at the age of thirty-eight, he was full of it, running, never shirking a tackle, he loved it. In goal we had Brad, who was Man of the Match that day, stopped everything. He was a great keeper. One of the best in the country, without a doubt.

With Brad playing so well, we grew in confidence and with twenty minutes left, the ball broke for me in the box. It bounced. I had to adjust my feet, but steered a deft finish past Neil Sullivan in their goal. It was a sweet moment. A finish I was proud of, a clever finish, but more importantly, it won us the League Cup and our fans had a day out to remember.

They could also soon celebrate our Premier League survival. To be fair, in the end we did more than merely survive. With the cup win behind us, we won half of our last dozen league games, finishing mid-table. I managed thirteen goals in the half-season I was there, a figure I was more than proud of, and I was, despite the issues at the training ground, eager to get going for the following campaign.

Such eagerness was validated. We had a top season, finishing sixth in the league and reaching the semi-final in our defence of the League Cup. Manchester United beat us in that match, and by now returning to Old Trafford with me as my team-mate was Dwight Yorke.

Dwight had been struggling at Manchester United. He was nowhere near the team and, like me, wanted first-team football. It was a pleasure to have him with us at Rovers. Graeme could be quite hard on the two of us. That's fine. He'd later say he didn't want us to drop our standards, but that was never a worry. For me, the big worry was my relationship with the manager, a relationship that had gone downhill, and quickly.

There were the usual issues. The continued involvement in training matches drove me potty, as did the now petty remarks about me and any success I had enjoyed. 'You're a myth,' he liked to say as our relationship soured with every working day. I wasn't going to keep quiet.

Those games in training were supposed to be intense, but with his constant involvement they were being slowed down. 'Boss, no disrespect, but you aren't playing on Saturday and this game is too stop-start. Why don't we get one of the kids over to join in?' It was input he clearly didn't appreciate or want to listen to.

One day we were working in the box. Quick one-touch passes with a defender or two in the middle. Graeme liked to stitch people up. He'd drop his pass in short, but then say, 'I can't go in the middle, I'm over fifty.' That used to make my blood boil. One day, I cracked. 'Get out, then. If you can't go in the middle, why are you joining in?'

He then dropped one short for me. 'Get in the middle,' he said.

'No.' The red mist – that old red mist – was descending.

'What?'

He went off in a mad tizz, calling me all sorts, repeating all that nonsense about me being a myth. I had had enough.

My inner voice was saying, 'Andrew, this is it. This has been brewing for months, and at some point you're probably going to get sacked anyway. We're near rock bottom, so stuff it.' When Graeme and I had first talked about me signing, I left that initial meeting thinking, 'Why not?' Now I was thinking about fighting him and the same question was firmly in my mind.

I started to march towards him, 'Let's have this tear-up,' but before I could get there three team-mates were on me. I was going ballistic. I had had enough! 'Leave it, Coley!' It wasn't the first time I'd heard team-mates saying that, but I wasn't listening. I wanted to get to him, but with the likes of Craig Short holding me back, it wasn't going to happen.

'Get inside,' Graeme shouted, 'training is over for you today.'

That made me laugh. Like I was going to stay outside there with him. I was dropped for the next game, but the problem was I really didn't care by this point. He was going to make life very hard for me, but for now I just didn't care.

*

Things got petty. He had me train with the kids. He had me in when the lads had a day off. He'd bring me on for the last minute of games just to humiliate me. I did not give a toss. All I knew was that he wouldn't break me. I could go back to my time in the game as a kid and draw strength from those experiences, knowing what football could be like, knowing how it works.

I also knew my rights. I was entitled to full training sessions. Too often I was training virtually alone, and that was enough to approach the Professional Footballers' Association. The name-calling and victimisation was one thing, but I wasn't being put to work and that wasn't on. I went to Bobby Barnes at the PFA hoping to get union advice and maybe some action. I was wrong. Instead, I got an old boys' network. I was disappointed. Gordon Taylor said he had too much respect for us both to truly get involved, but he was my union head, not Graeme's. I was the player here. At least look into it. Instead, I dropped it and chose to ride it out, always knowing something might blow up between us at any moment.

Funnily enough, it was an incident with Yorkey that heightened things and probably hastened my departure. It seemed Graeme was wary of me and Dwight. We'd played well for him, continued to score goals for him, but as time passed and relationships broke down, he became more cutting. He had two good, young strikers: Paul Gallagher and Jon Stead. He would play them off us, telling everyone that these two were the real deal, the future of the club, trying to get a rise out of us.

I liked Paul and Jon, no problem there, but it was all the grandstanding, Graeme's constant need to show everyone who was boss, that was the issue. He was always trying to take me down a peg or two. That didn't stop.

One day, in training, the same old issues. He was playing in a game with us but he left one right on Yorkey. It was a naughty challenge. Like those towards the end of his playing days. Yorkey had a very deep gash on his shin. He rolled up his sock, and there was the Dwight smile. 'OK, it's like that, is it?' he said. 'Let's play.'

So we played, and then it happened. There are times in games when you get the perfect scenario. The ball sits up and it is in just the right place – the right place to be won, but also the right place to half do someone. The ball was in that place, between player and manager, and Dwight absolutely launched Graeme, I mean launched him. It was like a cartoon, with Graeme going up and up, before, crash, he hit the ground with a thump and lost it. The session was over. 'Everyone get in.' Dwight was pleading innocence, that smile still on his face.

I was in the shower when I heard a commotion and someone ran in, saying Dwight had lost it. I had never known him to lose his temper, but apparently the argument had continued in front of the chief executive, John Williams, until Dwight had left.

John knew things were getting out of hand. Dwight and Graeme were one thing, but with the continued bad blood between me and the manager and the atmosphere around the place, something had to give. It was me or Graeme, and I understood it had to be me.

Things didn't get any better and one night I phoned John. I explained that it could go off at any time and it would make Dwight's run-in with him look like a kids' picnic. He didn't want the bad press that the sacking of a senior pro would bring the club, and he wasn't going to sack Graeme. I was almost due a loyalty bonus for the three seasons I'd been there but I couldn't have cared less about that. I wasn't going to hang around there for some bonus. No, it was time to leave.

It was a time of huge frustration for me. I so wanted to see out my career at Blackburn Rovers. That picture in my head had seemed so perfect – great club, family club, great team, scoring goals, still achieving things – but it had gone. Three years at the top level there and then maybe bow out. That was no longer possible.

Instead, I was left scratching. Scratching for a new home, the right place to call it a day, a new picture. I would, of course, keep looking, but that picture was no longer as clear.

Leaving Manchester United had been hard. Only with hindsight do I see it as the one single regret of my long career, but it showed we never know what is around the corner. Today, for all the trouble we caused each other, I bear no ill will against Graeme Souness. Since retiring from the game, I have been through so much. A serious illness cares little for the medals I've won, but it has taught me about empathy.

I now understand that you have to see both sides of a story. Graeme is a man with his own life, his own issues and even his own health concerns. In 2016, I was working for BeIN Sports on the World Cup with Richard Keys and Andy Gray. The guys would ask me if I had a problem with Graeme and I said no. I wasn't lying. He was also working there and one night I ran into him in the hotel corridor. Just me and him.

'Coley,' he said. 'I'd like to apologise.'

I was shocked.

'I'd like to say sorry for what went on at Rovers.'

I had nothing but admiration for him and walked away understanding further that football can be a very strange place to work, and that we run into so many different people along the way, with their own back-stories. As I walked away from Ewood Park in the summer of 2004, my journey wasn't over yet. My search for a final home continued.

13

HAVE BOOTS, WILL TRAVEL

I just wanted to be happy somewhere.

I really appreciate my career. How could I not? Settled and successful during arguably the most extraordinary era in the history of the most extraordinary football club. A Manchester United player, my family happy, financially secure, able to get out of bed in the morning smiling, excited about the day and working with the best in the business.

This football business that we all love can be a crazy place, though. I knew that from a young age. As a young man, I had stepped down to step up, leaving a giant in Arsenal and playing my football in the third and second tiers with Fulham and Bristol City respectively. I knew how the whole game worked. If, as a young apprentice, I had been wrapped up in cotton wool at Highbury, I had shredded it since then, and now understood that football is so much more than television and trophies.

For many looking in, that's how it seems. Especially today. All glitz and glamour. Football is like a swan and the superstars at the super-clubs are the elegant white feathers, all beauty and poise. Look under the surface, though, and you'll see the graft, the search for a living, the uncertainty that is the experience of so many footballers trying to make their way.

These are the players who live insecure lives. Driving miles to train, chasing agents who have better things to do, moving from club to club, from town to town, missing their kids, convincing their wives that soon they'll be settled, listening to promises from managers, putting up with lies, accepting short contracts or uncertain loans, hoping that the next move will be the one.

The months immediately after I left Arsenal had opened my eyes to that side of football, but for the last four years of my career I lived it. I was lucky, I had made a few quid, so I won't suggest I had those kind of worries, but I understand the nomadic life of a footballer trying to find a home. After Blackburn, seven clubs, in a little over four seasons. A whirlwind life, taking me from one corner of the country to another, cherishing phone calls with the kids that I didn't see, all because I wanted to finish in the right way, all because I wanted to be happy somewhere.

Like most things in football, it started with a phone call. It was Lee Clark. My old mate Clarky was now at Fulham, and just as he had been keen for me join Newcastle when I was at Bristol City, now he was telling me I should join his team. I was interested. Shirley and I had talked about moving to London when Devante had finished his primary school, but Fulham were doing well – I could move now and get it started and then the family could join me when the time was right.

I met the manager, Chris Coleman, or Cookie as he is known, and I liked him. Cookie is the most jovial man. His own career was cut short by injury but he was so enthusiastic about the game, and about footballers. He got us.

We went away on tour and had a night out, and rather than moaning at us all and punishing us, he put training back a couple of hours. That might sound like pandering to players, but it isn't. It was pre-season, we were bonding, he understood how players behaved, and when we did train, the sessions were excellent.

He would analyse opponents, he would prepare a team for a particular weekend. That was very fresh back then, close to how coaches work today. I was impressed with everything Cookie did, and the club when I joined was a buzzing, happy place, and that was mainly down to the manager and his coaching staff.

Money helped too. The club I had joined on loan in the early 1990s no longer existed. Fulham was now a Premier League set-up. A few bob had been put into every aspect of the place and that was most evident when you looked around the dressing room.

Edwin van der Sar in goal, Clarky in midfield, good overseas players such as Steed Malbranque and Luís Boa Morte. It was a solid and talented group. Decent young-sters such as Zat Knight, who should have gone further in the game, and Collins John, a Dutch striker who was the greatest forward in the world – according to him.

My old mate Leroy Rosenior's boy was there too. That'll make you feel old. Liam was great. He gravitated towards me, and was always wanting to learn about the game. Leroy had been so helpful to me when I was starting out and it was nice to help Liam. You come across some senior pros who are a little bitter – I certainly had – and distant, unwilling to help, jealous. I never understood that, and I would take any chance I got to chat about the game with the youngsters at any club at which I worked.

Talking to the kids was another reminder that I missed my own. When I signed for Fulham and moved to London, I'll be honest, I didn't appreciate just how much I'd miss my children. Cookie understood my predicament – I would have the odd day off, if we played up north I would stay over – but it's not enough. Not when you've been used to being there, waking up with them and putting them to bed.

If I was missing my kids at home, on the pitch, I

wasn't often missing the target. I got thirteen goals for Fulham in the 2004–05 season. We played a nice brand of football, chances were always going to be limited, but despite being almost thirty-four, I always backed myself. Players today who get into double figures can go for £40 million or so, so my free transfer to south-west London looked a decent deal.

We did OK. Mid-table. The football was always attractive, but we probably lacked a bit of needle. Players who, when it got a bit tasty, rolled up their sleeves and said, 'Let's have it.' We were a bit too nice, but I liked playing for Cookie and for the club, at least I did until missing my children began to affect my football.

I wasn't myself. I had family and friends in London, but something was missing and that was day-to-day contact with Devante and Faith. I again suggested to Shirley that they all move down, but once again she was adamant that their school came first. I understood and I didn't want to push it, and so my mind started to drift towards me moving back.

I went to Cookie, and as ever he was easy to talk to. He listened to me and understood my predicament. I had a two-year contract, so he wanted to find a replacement, but it was decided that, after one season, I was going home, and at first it looked like my next location would be a familiar one.

*

Blackburn Rovers were the first in for me. Mark Hughes was by now manager and with all the respect I had for him, and my fondness for the club itself, it meant I was well up for it. All the numbers looked good, Fulham wanted a bit of cash for me but not much, but soon the talks went quiet. Rovers had bought Craig Bellamy for a lot of money, but I was excited about that. Bellers was a top player, sprightly, rapid – he could do all my running! This could be interesting.

Sparky called me, though, and it wasn't happening. He said his budget had gone on Bellamy, and that he couldn't make the numbers work. I was not happy. It had been perfect. With my home situation, my options were limited. I needed a new club, but I needed that new club to be in the north-west.

And then Manchester City came in for me. The blue half of the city in which I had enjoyed so much success. I'll be honest, my legacy at Old Trafford crossed my mind. What would the United fans think? How would the City fans take to me? These thoughts run through your mind, but I broke it down and one name came to me: Denis Law.

Now, I am not saying I am anything like Denis, a player some would argue is the best ever to play for Manchester United. But, like him, I had a great rapport with the United faithful and I thought that if I got it right, that relationship, like Denis's, needn't suffer. A more recent example might have put me off. Peter Schmeichel had slightly blotted his image with the fans, for what some punters saw as an overly zealous celebration of a City goal against United, but I believed, or hoped, that I could be more Denis than Peter.

The Manchester City I signed for in 2005 was a world away from the gold-plated Taj Mahal that we know in modern times. The place was run on shirt buttons. Everything was on a budget, the chairman was old-school, a guy called John Wardle, a local busi-nessman. The manager was my old England team-mate Stuart Pearce. When we met, he quickly reminded me about the day I stood up to him. 'Psycho', as he was known, was playing centre-back for Newcastle when I faced him, and at one point he shouted at his partner, 'Knock his ******* block off.' I stopped and said, 'Never mind *him* knocking my block off, why don't *you* do it?'

The club were away on pre-season in Thailand when I signed. I joined up with them and was apprehensive. You often are walking into a new squad, but I had the whole United thing in my head. Ten minutes into my first lunch with the lads, I was almost on the floor laughing. There I was breaking bread with new team-mates and suddenly, Spider-Man came rolling into the room. I say Spider-Man, it was someone in an outfit about six sizes too small for him, the mask and everything.

'Who the hell is that?' I was thinking as this character rolled around the floor.

The whole room was in hysterics, before eventually the mask came off to reveal the left-back Ben Thatcher. Ben was so funny, had a bit of a reputation, and might not have been the full ticket, but from that moment he always had me in stitches.

I also knew Trevor Sinclair. Trevor had been at Lilleshall with me, in the year below.

'Bloody hell, Coley,' he said, when I arrived. 'You were horrible to me as a kid.'

'What?'

'You were a nightmare, mate. You never stopped bullying me.'

I explained that we had got the same treatment from the boys above us and just passed it down. We laughed about it and it was nice to have a familiar face.

There were others I knew. David James in goal, Robbie Fowler; further quality in Sylvain Distin; good youngsters in Micah Richards, Stephen Ireland and Joey Barton. On that tour in Thailand, Joey had had a fight with big Richard Dunne, but I have to say, he was never a problem with me. Different yes, lively yes, but a good young footballer wanting to learn. I got on well with him.

Darius Vassell was there too, who I knew a bit. Vass was a fine young player and we formed a good partnership at City. He was my legs, full of running. He later said I was the best player he ever played with, which was nice to hear. To be playing with great potential like Vass, to be scoring with him while helping him, that was exactly what I was looking for in my final years.

Ben Thatcher used to give me loads of stick. 'Oi, Coley, you old ****,' he'd say by way of a greeting. 'Are you dyeing your hair? You must be, you don't have a grey one, and what are you? Fifty-six?' It was all good-natured and he always made me smile. 'Oi, Coley, you're out of order, making Vass do all your running for you,' was another one.

Yes, I was happy in my first months at the Etihad, but just weeks in, standing alongside Manchester United players in the tunnel at Old Trafford before an early-season derby, I felt anxious. This was Old Trafford. I was in blue. How would the fans who once sang my name react to my return? What if they booed me? That would have been hard to take.

Fortunately, I got a good reception. We drew 1–1, and we actually beat United at the Etihad 3–1 later in the campaign, proving what a decent side we were. Unfortunately, I got injured in March, my knee. I had nicked the cartilage and needed a small op. I expected to be back in a month, no more than six weeks, in time for the last games of the season.

The club sent me to a so-called specialist in the north-west and as soon as I walked in I had my doubts about the place. As I say, the club was run on a tight budget, but I was there and had the op, and soon my fears were realised. During my rehab, every time I worked on the knee it blew up like a balloon.

It wasn't right. The physio at the club could see that and recommended another look. This time I took myself to Andy Williams, the top knee man in London, and he found they had left a floating piece of bone on the knee. I was furious. I needed another operation and instead of five weeks, I was out for three months. It proved to be the end of me at the club.

That summer I took the family to Sandy Lane in Barbados. Pure relaxation after the operation. A million miles away from the hustle and bustle of my day job. Or so I thought. Who was there, sharing the pool and the cocktail bar, but Portsmouth manager Harry Redknapp and his wife, Sandra. I had met Harry a few times, but didn't know him well. We said our hellos.

For the next few days, I'd be by the pool and Harry would pass by and sit on the lounger next to me. Nothing but small talk.

'All right, son,' he'd say. 'Nice 'ere, innit?'

'Oh, it's lovely, Harry.'

Then it would be 'How's it goin', son?'

'All good, Harry, thanks. You?'

'Yeah, triffic.'

Or 'What a beautiful day, Coley. Family enjoyin' it?'

'Oh, they love it, thanks, Harry.'

One day, he joined me and said, 'Listen, how do you fancy joining Portsmouth, son?'

I guess that was the end of the small talk. I had to explain that I had an offer on the table of another year at City, that my family were settled up there. 'We'll give you two years,' he said. Now, that was interesting. I could go back to City and say another club were offering an extra season. Nice to have collateral in this game. Let's see what they say.

When I returned, City wouldn't budge. They cited my age, the knee injury too. The money man, Alistair Mackintosh, was adamant and wouldn't budge and so I had another decision to make. I went to Shirley. Portsmouth had supposedly come into money, through the Israeli businessman Alexandre Gaydamak, and were going to have a go at it.

Decent wages, an extra year on offer, more security, the promise of football. Two more years and then that will be it, I'll pack it in. There was the problem of me missing the family again, but this time Shirley agreed we should all make the move and so it looked as if Hampshire was going to be my final destination.

We bought a new home near Southampton and began a new life. Portsmouth were trying to do the same. They were laying grand and expensive foundations. Joining me there for the 2006–07 season were Sol Campbell and Lauren from Arsenal, Niko Kranjčar, Glen Johnson (on loan from Chelsea), David James, Kanu – big, big names.

It was a good squad and I looked forward to getting going. The only thing was, the patter I had heard from Harry about me playing games, the big talk about being part of his plans, none of it was true. Not one iota. Nothing he said materialised, and it wasn't long before I was pulling my hair out. Harry preferred Benjani and Kanu. Fine, but I wasn't even tried. It wasn't like we were winning every game, but I had to watch from the sidelines, grabbing short bursts of action, unable to get into a rhythm and unable to stay patient.

I was doing my nut. I became a nightmare to be around. When senior pros aren't playing they quickly become grumpy old men and that was me. It must have been horrible living with me. Faith was struggling to settle in at her new school and missed her pals up north. Devante was at Southampton's academy and they looked after him, but he too struggled with a new school. Shirley was restless because it wasn't working out, and

I was thinking to myself, 'Why have I disrupted my whole family for this?'

Eventually Shirley and the kids moved back to Cheshire. I was left knocking about an empty house that I'd put back on the market, missing them again and wondering why I had bothered, why I had listened to Harry's spiel. In March 2007, Steve Bruce got in touch and I was off to Birmingham City in the Championship on loan. All I wanted was a chance to play football. Harry couldn't get his head around why I had dropped a division. 'Why has he gone?' he asked Sol Campbell. The Sol man simply told him that I wanted to get a game.

So, now I was driving to Birmingham from Cheshire for training, which wasn't ideal, but at least I was playing. Birmingham were pushing for promotion and Brucie said that if we got promoted they'd make the move permanent. Sorted. Birmingham did get promoted, but was the move permanent? No. Another broken promise and I was back at Portsmouth. Back to square one. This is what the life of a footballer can too often entail. Thoughts of packing it in were close, of course, but there was too strong a feeling for the game, and the fact that I knew I could still offer a team something.

*

Harry clearly thought otherwise. That summer, in pre-season, Portsmouth were off to play in the Asia Cup. The manager told me not to come. He gave me some excuse about my fitness, but I had had enough. Time to have it out properly. He had convinced me that I was going to be part of his plans and then not played me, he had mugged me off. Now he was giving me some nonsense about my legs. Was it too much to ask for an honest manager who just told me the truth?

The team went off to Asia and I was left to train at home. I hadn't moved back to the south coast. Sod that. Every morning and every afternoon there was a shuttle flight between Manchester and Southampton, so I was on that. Tiring, long, but what else could I do? There were days I would wake up and think, 'I'm not going in,' but I always did. I might have to leave early to get the flight home, but by then no one at the club cared. On his return, Harry and I had it out again, and he agreed to pay me up for my contract and I could leave the whole waste of time behind.

So with the 2007–08 season starting soon, I was at home, not even kicking my heels, just chilling, when the phone went: 'Hey, Coley, it's Roy here, what are you up to?' Roy Keane was now manager at Sunderland in the Premier League.

'Just taking it easy, Schiz,' I said.

'Come and have a chat.'

Roy and I had that chat and it was great. An honest chat between two old friends. No skulduggery. I trusted him, he knew what he'd get from me, and so I signed for Sunderland. I have to say I really enjoyed being there. I didn't play as much as I wanted because of niggly injuries, but it was a great environment. Yorkey was there too, which helped, but they were a good group of lads, good young players who wanted to learn from us, and frankly it was fascinating to watch Skip (I now called him Skip, as 'Schiz' was never going to work for my manager) try his luck at management.

He hadn't changed a bit from our United days. I had so much respect for him as a player, and as the boss he was exactly the same. I could never say a bad word about Roy, but I did wonder if that could work. He demanded so much from his team-mates as a player, but as a manager, those demands, when working with lesser players, aren't always realised.

His fiery temper certainly hadn't diminished at all. One day we went to Everton and got pumped 7–1. I wasn't playing but I was in the dressing room afterwards, not a place for the faint of heart. Skip walked in with this look on his face, an expression of pure anger. He got started and built gradually, cranking it up from a bollocking to a nuclear explosion. Paint was peeling off the wall as he laid into everyone individually, before I felt I had to step in.

'OK, Skip, that's enough now.' And it was. They knew they had played badly and I like to believe that Roy had enough respect for me to know I wasn't butting in, but giving good advice. The scoreline told the players how poorly they had played. Time to get out of there and move on.

Injury further hindered my appearances but when I returned to fitness, I still had that desire to play the game. Getting into Roy's team regularly wasn't going to happen right then and so another loan deal cropped up in the second half of the season, this time with Burnley, back in the Championship. Money had nothing to do with things, I just wanted to play, and Roy understood that, even telling me he took his hat off to me for my decision to join Owen Coyle's side.

Owen was like a big kid. All enthusiasm. Training was a buzz, all kinds of games – hit the crossbar, get the ball, dribble it back, put it between the legs of your team-mate, all sorts. I liked him a lot, he reminded me of Kevin Keegan in my early days at Newcastle, and I got on with playing and trying to score some goals.

One day, against Queens Park Rangers, I got three. Any hat-trick is a lift, but on this occasion not only did I get a standing ovation from the Rangers fans, but when I got back to the coach and switched on my phone, the first message I got was from Roy: 'Brilliant hat-trick, Coley!' He could have dismissed it. It was a classy touch from a very good friend.

Burnley missed out on promotion that year and I missed out on a permanent move to Turf Moor. Was this it? Thoughts of finishing were very real now. But then one last offer. I couldn't help myself. One last fling. This time at Nottingham Forest. It looked perfect. Going back to Nottingham. Perfect symmetry.

The thing is, I had left Nottingham at fourteen and didn't see it as home any more. Yes, my parents lived there, and my brother and three sisters, but if there was any sentimentality about the decision to sign, it was from my late grandad Vincent, a man who had missed pretty much all I had achieved in the game and who had always said, thanks to that love for Brian Clough, that I had to play for Forest.

I used the word 'sentimentality' there, and that leads me to my relationship with my agent, Paul Stretford. For all my running around between the clubs of England, Paul had become more and more distant from me. He did a few of the deals, including the one at Sunderland, but phone calls were starting to be ignored, texts not returned, and that was odd.

I had been with Paul since the day I signed for Newcastle. We had had a rolling contract since then, but he had become so much more than an agent. He was my mate. As the years rolled by, he had me to stay in his home when I was building a new house. I could sit with him and talk about my life, my worries, my hopes. He was there for advice. I was there for him too. I trusted him and I had never found that easy with anyone. I trusted him so much that he is godfather to Devante.

And then, not long after I left Portsmouth, he started to pull away and I began to wonder why. Had I done something wrong? Then a conversation I had had with an old Newcastle team-mate came back to me. Scott Sellars had initially recommended Paul to me, but then years later he had taken me to one side. 'Coley,' he said. 'There will come a point in your life when Stretford does not need you any more and he will discard you like he did me.'

I wasn't having it at the time. My relationship with Paul was different. Loads of players fell out with agents and went their separate ways, but that's the thing, we were more than player and agent. This was closer. Scott couldn't be right. Could he?

Before I went to Forest in 2008, clearly my last move, I caught up with Paul and we had a meeting. We sat down, the atmosphere a bit tense. I told him I wanted to play for one more season, and then we could think about what I'd do next. He looked sheepish and then he said it.

'Andrew, there is nothing more I can do for you.'

The words hung in the air. 'Excuse me?' He repeated it and I lost it. This was a man who had shared so much of my life, was close to my family, and now he was treating me like some other mug, talking to me like I was some sort of dog, ready to be put down. I wanted to tear into him but he was unmoved. He was basically saying, 'Goodbye, thanks for everything but that's that.' It was cold and it hurt. We have hardly spoken since.

I still had some football to play. Any sentimental feelings I had about playing at the City Ground were quickly erased, though, as I realised the club was operating under a cloud of politics. Colin Calderwood was manager, but half picking the team was clearly the chairman, Nigel Doughty. I won't talk ill of the dead, but I'm sure he was pulling the strings in the dressing room.

One midweek game we played at Sheffield Wednesday. We lost, but I played decent. In training on the Friday I noticed Colin circling around me. It was like a shark fin in a movie. 'If you have something to say, then say it,' I was thinking, before finally he pulled me to one side and spat it out. 'Coley, I'm leaving you out on Saturday.' He followed it up with something about my legs looking like they'd gone, but he hadn't taken me off when we needed a goal in Sheffield.

I thought it was nonsense, but I'd had enough. What was I chasing? I was done and I told him so. All this battling, for what? I didn't even go to the game on the Saturday, and on the Monday the chief executive, Mark Arthur, approached me and said the club were looking to terminate my contract. I wanted to laugh in his face. 'Hold on, but I told Colin on Friday I was finished.'

I knew what was happening, they wanted to look like they were in control, that they had the power. I told him that I knew how this club was run, that it was going nowhere in a hurry and I was off. I walked out, no boots in my hand, nothing, just the proud knowledge that when it came to it, I was in control of my retirement, not some chief executive. I made the announcement immediately, which must have annoyed Forest, and that was that. October 2008 and I had retired. I had come into the game fighting, and I left it the same way.

And then suddenly, you're no longer a footballer. It's weird. I was pleased to be out of all the hassle, the rubbish that the last four seasons had shown me, but you do quickly mourn your career. The banter, the dressing room, all of that, but you also miss the structure. You know where you need to be when you're a footballer, you know what you have to wear. It's funny, but when that structure disappears from your life, you're suddenly at a loose end.

I had time to look back at my career. I was proud of it. I remembered Paul Davis, my old Arsenal team-mate, saying, 'You've always done it your way,' and I guess he was right. I half laugh at the situations I got myself into at times, but my record, the third top scorer in Premier League history, is there in black and white. I'd won the lot. Played with and against the most incredible people. I may have fallen out with a few of them along the way, but I made far more friends than I lost. Little did I know that soon, friends and people would mean more than any winners' medal.

14

I'VE GOT A LITTLE PROBLEM

I am smiling. A rare thing on a face that for a number of years hasn't been used to such optimism. I'm in Hanoi City, it's 2015. The hustle and bustle is energising, the lovely people have their own grins that eagerly greet mine. The city alone is enough to awaken the darkest of moods. Modern buildings mixed with age-old history. Colours everywhere. Reds, yellows, pinks; green vines that climb the walls as if wanting a better view. Motorbikes swerve past their pedalled cousins, hooting as they go, while markets sell food and trinkets to a never-ending crowd.

I love it. I am in Vietnam with Manchester United in my role as a club ambassador, meeting sponsors and partners. I have to admit it's nice to be away. Nice to smile. Nice to be somewhere new, somewhere so pretty.

It's so different from life at home. For four years our lives have been in turmoil. Faith has become ill and, seeing a child in distress, so seriously ill, nothing can prepare you for it, nothing in your character suggests you'll be able to handle it. I played top-flight football, challenged myself to go up against the very best footballers on the planet, refused to accept defeat so many times on a football pitch, but when you are faced with your child's mortality, you wonder if you have the strength to cope.

As I walk around Hanoi smiling, it dawns on me just how hard life has become. By now, Faith is getting better, dealing with her illness in the most inspiring of ways, but it has been a hard, dark time. Little do I know, though, as I gaze around at my exciting temporary surroundings, that my problems are far from over.

After I had retired, there was the typical period of not knowing what to do with myself. I remember one morning Shirley coming to me with a stern face. I was lying on the sofa just chilling out.

'What are you doing?' she said.

'Not a lot.'

'Well, you'd better do something soon, because I have my own routine, and I want you out from under my feet.'

It was a shock, if I'm honest, but she was right, I had to think about my next move.

I took up golf, and I enjoyed it, getting down to 12, but it wasn't enough. Then, in 2009, I got a call from one of the girls at Manchester United asking if I'd be interested in doing some corporate work. At first, I wasn't having it. Meeting people, talking about past glories. It wasn't for me. I had always thought that, having retired, I wouldn't want to wallow in what I had done as a footballer, and this seemed to be doing exactly that.

'Just give it a go,' she said. 'If you don't like it after a while, give it up.'

Why not, I thought, and as I got into it, working on match days, doing corporate events, learning more about the other side of the game, the sponsorship and part-nerships, meeting fantastic people from all over the world and travelling, I grew to love it. But then our lives were turned upside down.

In 2011, my daughter, Faith, was ten. She was such a happy kid, but she had had the odd health issue as a younger child – arthritis in her knee, a problem with her eye too – so we were always on the look-out, and therefore when she was sent home from school with increasing regularity, we began to be more and more concerned. One day, my brother had come up to see me for lunch, when Shirley called to say that I needed to pick Faith up from school, as once again she wasn't well.

I remember getting her to the car, and there was nothing to her. She seemed so weak. My brother, Des, took one look at her and said, 'She doesn't look right.'

I had seen her ill before but this was different, and because it had been going on for a bit, I decided to make a call.

Phil Batty had been my doctor at Old Trafford and Blackburn Rovers. We had always got on, so I phoned him and explained that Faith wasn't right and asked if he could arrange for someone to see her. I didn't like using my footballing connections, but I needed something quick and Phil came through, getting us in to see someone at the Bridgewater Hospital in Manchester. They ran some tests and sent us home, where Shirley and I went to bed feeling better that she'd been checked out.

And then, horror. We woke up, turned on our phones and we were greeted with a message from Phil that said, 'Get Faith to the hospital as quickly as you can.' Boom. It was like a sledgehammer. We rushed her in and discovered that Faith's blood count was down to two, when a healthy child's should be at around twelve.

Like so many fathers and daughters, there has always been an incredible bond between Faith and me. There is something so special about the relationship, so pure. Then I saw her on a hospital bed, surrounded by busy medical staff, knowing that soon she would be full of tubes, having blood transfused into her fragile little veins. I won't lie, as I walked into that room, I folded.

In football, words like 'coward' are thrown around.

Shirk a challenge, succumb to an injury or even miss a penalty, you're a coward. It's normal to be labelled. Part of the game. As a player, I would give it back to anyone who called me that. I wasn't having it, but now as I walked into that hospital room and saw Faith, I don't care what people want to call me, I folded.

I was on the floor. All I wanted was to swap places with her, to give her my strength, but for that moment I had none of my own and I collapsed into the door. Throughout my life, I have not been able to cope with the death or illness of loved ones. My own illness and injuries while playing football were one thing, I could personalise that and do things my way, but when those I love have been affected, I have always struggled.

My grandad Vincent, my brother-in-law Donovan, who was like a brother to me, when they both died, I had found it so hard to talk about, and instead I would internalise it all, keeping my feelings in, hiding any emotion and not wanting to talk about loss. Now it was happening in front of me to the most precious person in my life. How was I going to manage myself and my family?

In my head I had a million and one questions. What can I do? What could I have done better? I wasn't coming up with any answers. As her treatment progressed, I was trying to cope, but it was internal and not always rational. Take the time I was in the hospital with Faith while she had a biopsy. I was holding her as a doctor cut into her, and she was crying, 'Daddy, please make it stop.' I just wanted to fill the doctor in, one punch and I could make it stop. That's all I could think. I couldn't rationally handle what Faith was going through and I found it harder and harder to be at the hospital for the week she was in. It was a place where all I could do was be the blubbering father. I wish I could have been stronger, but watching her go through tests, seeing her in pain, it threw me in ways I can't explain.

It was at home that I thought I could be positive, but that brought its own problems, as it was clear that Shirley and I were coping in very different ways. Shirley wanted to deal with worst-case scenarios. I saw those as negatives. Maybe it's my sporting past, but if I was ever told I'd be out for months, it would all be about getting back in weeks. Shirley was all about preparation, wanting to talk about the 'what ifs', and I would draw away from that, and therefore from her.

'What if that treatment doesn't work?' she'd ask. Or, 'What if she gets worse?'

I wasn't having it. I couldn't get involved in all that. 'We'll move to a country where the treatment will work,' I'd say, or, 'She won't get worse, our Faith will be back just like before, running around, smiling.'

There is no right or wrong. We both loved her so

much. It was just two caring parents coping differently, but ultimately it was breaking the relationship. Shirley resented the way I handled our daughter's illness. It was such a hard time. Faith had so many tests and blood transfusions. In time, they would diagnose a disorder with her bone marrow and lupus, a disease that attacks the immune system. She copes with it so well, so admirably, even writing blogs about her health, wanting to help others, and I am so proud of her and the way she dealt with things.

What is clear, though, is that the experience drove a wedge between Shirley and me. We had been together since we were teenagers. We'd had our ups and downs like any married couple, but we'd also had good times, her support vital to me for so long, and we had two wonderful kids. But now we were at loggerheads about our daughter's illness and treatments.

'You weren't there for me,' was something she would often say. Yes, I had struggled to be at the hospital every day for that first week, but my input, my positivity at home, that's how I had wanted to help my family. With that gap between us becoming a chasm, I retreated further into myself – unable to engage with my wife, knowing that we would only fight, and instead battling with it all myself. Negative voices in my head (louder than the ones I heard as an insecure footballer) were constant.

Was I a good enough husband or father? I knew my wife resented me, I had doubts, every day, and to cope I became more and more silent at home. I was in pain. Have I let my family down? Something in me died when Faith was ill, but over time I have tried to look at things differently. I want no praise, but I can be positive, knowing that the phone call I made to Phil Batty that day and the instant treatment I got for my daughter probably saved her life.

In that period, I was being judged at home by my wife for my initial response to Faith being in hospital. Maybe I could have coped differently, but who can say how such a trauma will affect a person? I felt that I deserved to be judged for the man she had always known. Instead, we were drifting apart, and while our daughter was fixing herself and coping, our marriage was doing the exact opposite.

With Faith getting better, I threw myself into work. I embraced my new role at Old Trafford, revelling in how it occupied my mind, embracing the normality of the day-to-day. I actually got more and more into the corporate side of things at the club. I enjoyed the trips away, probably appreciating being away from the tension at home, and so when I was asked to go to Vietnam in 2015, I jumped at the chance.

I loved Vietnam and its vibrancy. When it was time to fly home, I packed my bag in my hotel room, thinking about what a fun and interesting trip it had been. Bags packed, I went to the loo and my pee smelt rancid. 'You need to drink more water, son,' I thought as I left for the airport.

When I arrived home I was exhausted. I felt ill, but I put it down to the long-haul flight and, typically for me when a bit under the weather, I took a couple of paracetamol and got into bed. Tomorrow was another day. No problem. But there was a problem.

The next day, still very tired, I was getting ready to go to dinner with Shirley and a couple of friends in a nice restaurant in Manchester. I put on a shirt and Shirley took one look at me and said, 'That shirt's too tight. You've put on weight in Asia.' I argued back, saying it was fine, but she was right. Just in the day since I got back, it seemed that I was bigger.

I had been obsessed with my weight when I retired. There was no way I was going to get big or lose my fitness, and so to hear my wife saying I'd put on weight, and so suddenly, did raise an eyebrow, but no problem, I'd work it off tomorrow. And so we went for dinner.

We were at our table and the dishes came and everyone tucked in. 'Mmmmmm, this is lovely,' they were all saying, but I was fuming because my food tasted of nothing. I was cursing. 'This food is rubbish, pass the salt and pepper, it is so bland.' They were all laughing at me, wondering why I was always so miserable. Again, I thought little of it, other than that it was the last time I'd be going to that place to eat.

The next day, I was sweating and feeling really bad. So tired, more weight was on, and Shirley was telling me to go to the doctor. Now, I come from a long line of men who don't go to doctors. We'll just take those paracetamol and it will all be OK. But as the day went on, I began to have my doubts. I still wasn't going to go to the doctor but I did call Mike Stone, an ex-Manchester United doctor. I explained my symptoms and he agreed to come over and see me.

He took a look and I could see he was thinking, 'What the hell is going on here?' The weight was so obvious and sudden, and he immediately got me an appointment at the Alexandra Hospital. They ran a few tests there, then I went home, where a friend was cooking for us, a meal that once again I cursed for its blandness, and I went to bed, still feeling far from OK.

Two days later, I got a call from Mike saying I needed to get myself to the Manchester Royal Infirmary, where a consultant would be waiting for me. 'OK, no problem, Mike. I have a few things to do later, but I'll pop by.' I drove into the hospital and remember not being in the mood for it all. I needed to be somewhere else soon, and while I didn't feel well, I thought I was wasting my time.

Mike Picton was the consultant and we got the small talk out of the way before he started to ask me questions. 'How did you get in?' he asked.

'I drove,' I replied, thinking this a strange question.

He started to ask more questions. I replied to each but I was irritable. *I have to be somewhere, can we hurry up?*

'You shouldn't have driven in,' he said.

You what? I'm thinking. Does he know how old I am? What does he mean I shouldn't have driven in? I'm a bit ill, not disabled. I was struggling with the questions – the usual issue with authority. A doctor telling me what I should and shouldn't do. I don't need this.

He told me he wanted to do a biopsy right now. Now? Well, I'm here, so OK, but I was still irritated by it all. They did the biopsy and then he said, 'You won't be going anywhere today, Andrew.'

'Are you mad? I have places to be.'

'Let's talk about your symptoms,' he says. 'How are your taste buds?'

I sat up. 'Yes, food has no taste.'

'How about going to the toilet?'

Suddenly it occurred to me that in the few days since I'd been back from Vietnam, I'd hardly been.

'Have you had hiccups?'

'No,' I said quickly, happy that he might be wrong.

'Itchy skin?'

'No, none of that.' I was feeling positive now, I was OK.

And then it happened. As we talked further, within less than half an hour, I had the hiccups and my skin felt like a million and one ants were crawling over it. I was sitting there, itching, hiccupping. Weight seemed to be piling on, right there in the room. I felt like Eddie Murphy in the *Nutty Professor* movies, and all the while I was starting to feel more and more ill.

Everything the consultant knew was going to happen was happening there and then – and suddenly I was in a bed. They were trying to find veins but having no joy. They tried my arm and my foot, before finally stabilising me, and while I was sedated, Mike talked to me. I was confused, but that was when I first heard the words 'kidney failure'.

There, in that hospital bed, it was being broken down for me, explained to me, but I wasn't taking it in. Due to a virus picked up in Vietnam, I had renal failure. The word 'failure' was hanging there. My stubbornness, a weakness and a strength in my life, wasn't having it. I was not that ill. There was no failure. Get me up and get me out of here.

Instead, within days, I was on dialysis. Shirley and

the kids had been informed and I told her specifically not to tell my parents. I didn't want them worrying about me until I was out of the hospital and knew more. From the day I had left home, aged just fourteen, to go to Lilleshall. I was very independent. I was supposed to look after myself, I certainly didn't want them seeing my strapped to a machine that was keeping me alive.

Dialysis is horrible. It's making you better, yes, but it is rank. You're on it for three or four hours, and then you are exhausted. In those days on dialysis, life was sleep. In the hospital, I would be constantly in and out of sleep. Visitors would sit at my bedside, watching me drift in and out of conversation. It was hard for them.

My life in football had probably saved me. The doctors told me that my physicality and the fact that I had remained fit helped me at first, but eventually my body had packed up, unable to take any more. If I hadn't got into hospital that day, with those toxins inside me, and if I had done the usual and gone to bed with two paracetamols, I would probably have died.

I know my son, Devante, struggled being at my bedside. He is like me. He might not admit it, but I could see he wasn't having it. There I was, his dad, a former footballer, athletic and strong. One minute I'm his hero and then suddenly I am weak – seventeen stone and vulnerable. Not even able to sit up and tell him it's all going to be OK.

My parents suffered too. Shirley had told them what was going on, despite my wishes, and to see them walk in the room and see me in bed, that was hard. My mum's face. 'Could this be it?' I could tell those thoughts were racing through her worried mind. She made conversation, brightened up the room as ever, but her eyes gave away her concerns.

My dad was no different. He sat next to me. Not talking. Silence, but in his eyes, you could see he was looking at his son, this kid he had fought with but never stopped loving in his way. He sat there and wondered if this was where it might end. Like me, there wasn't much coming out, but the turmoil inside was palpable.

So was the tension between Shirley and my dad. I have mentioned before that the two of them were like water and oil. When Shirley walked into the hospital room, my dad stood up and left without a hello. Shirley went mad at me. How could I let him be so rude? I was sick as a dog, huge, wired up. I was fighting for my life and had no strength to fight her. Shirley was, of course, brilliant while I was ill, looking after the kids, supporting me, but once again the cracks in our marriage were clear.

*

I was in hospital for two weeks before they let me leave. It was such a relief to be in my own home. Shirley took Faith away on holiday when I got back, a decision I found a bit strange considering my condition, but one I didn't argue about, especially as my nephew Alexander was staying with me, looking after me, making me laugh. Alex is the son of my oldest sister, Patsy. He was twenty-six then, and we were close, as I was with all my nephews.

With Alex looking after me, I went into hospital to have my lines put in. That involves them cutting you open and running wires over your collarbone (not a nice experience) and preparing you for emergency dialysis. I had the procedure, but later at home I felt even worse than usual. I was hallucinating. It turned out that the lines they ran through me were infected. It never rains, it pours!

The word 'transplant' was only being mentioned in passing. In my mind that was never going to happen. Ever. The medication would work and one day I would wake up from this nightmare, back to normal. In those dark, tired days, normal seemed so distant, but I tried my best to keep some connection with happier times.

I continued to go the gym, for instance. I couldn't do much, and when I got home all I could do was sleep, but even the briefest of work-outs meant I was fighting this. My weight was a clear problem. I had been photographed and Faith was getting asked questions about me at school. 'Look at the state of your dad!' and 'Who ate all the pies?' All of that. It was around then the BBC's *Football Focus* asked me to go on the show and, despite hating my large appearance and despite feeling dog rough, I knew I couldn't hide from the world. I was more than happy to talk about football, but the time was right to talk about my disease too.

Bang, loads of sympathy. While so many people had been quick to prejudge me, plenty more got in touch on Twitter, wanting to offer support and wanting to discuss their own illnesses. I was touched and communicated as well as I could, but I was still refusing to take it all seriously – I was soon going to be better.

Shirley wanted to talk about a harder future. She wanted to look at options, and those worst-case scenarios. She would talk about dialysis, she'd send me stuff to read on transplants, and I was just not having it. This time it was *my* illness. I refused to be dictated to about how we dealt with *my* illness. In my mind, all I'd got was a little problem, and soon it would be gone.

I understand why Shirley was frustrated. I understand how hard it was for her. She believed I should be preparing myself in a certain way. My thoughts were different. It might have been opposite to how she and the doctors saw things, but that was that. This was my illness and I couldn't handle it any other way. I had a little problem and soon I would beat it.

I was relying on my medication. Those pills. For now, they were my way out of all this, but soon they would turn on me too. The pills I had been on began to fail and the new lot sent me from a nightmare to hell. On them, I had nothing. No strength, no will to get up, nothing. I'd sit in front of the television with the kids and when not asleep, I'd cry for no reason. 'Are you OK, Dad?' I'd hear, but they'd get no reply. I remember just wanting to end myself. Something had to change, and soon the doctors were starting to say that word I hated more and more: TRANSPLANT.

To use a simple football analogy: for me, talk of a transplant was like being 1–0 down in a massive game, desperate to score the vital equaliser, but seeing the manager calling me off and being substituted. A transplant to me meant my number was up, that my body had lost, and I no longer had any real say in the result.

It was irrational, but so much in my mind was back then. Soon I would have to face up to reality. Seven months after my trip to Vietnam, and I was dog ill, on the floor, the meds taking as much from me as the kidney. 'OK,' I said finally. 'I'm ill.'

The doctor came to me and agreed. 'The drugs aren't working,' he declared. 'That's it, Andrew, you have to have a transplant. It's time to find a donor.'

I wasn't having it, but I knew my options were minimal. I still had this idea that soon I would wake up and things would be just like they were before. At home, I took so much inspiration from Faith. The two of us couldn't have been closer, but having become ill myself, we had an understanding. It's so hard for others to be there and say they know what you are going through. I couldn't truly do it to Faith when she was ill, but now we could look each other in the eyes and just get it. She could look at me on my lowest days and say, 'Dad, tomorrow will be better.' From her they were so much more than just comforting words.

My whole family were incredible. When it became clear that I needed a donor, they all stepped up. All of them. Sisters, brothers, nephews, cousins, my friends, everyone stepped up. Of course, I resisted the idea. If I had always hated letting loved ones down, I certainly wasn't going to be taking any major organs from them.

I was clinging to that idea of a sudden cure. I was so ill, though, I can't even remember if I truly believed it. By now I was sleeping fourteen or fifteen hours a day. I was a shell of a man. No energy, no strength.

On the rare occasions I was awake, my thoughts were sullen. One day, Alex came over to be with me. Alex and I had always enjoyed each other's company. Like me, he is a man of few words, and he was more than comfortable in my silence.

On this occasion, that was just as well, because as we sat on the sofa, I was out for the count. When I woke up, there he was, with a serious look on his face. He began to speak.

'Uncle,' he said.

'What's up, nephew?' I said groggily.

'I'm not having this any more. I won't sit around and see you like this any more, unc. You're having my kidney. I am doing this.'

There was a tone in his voice, a look in his eye, that suggested his mind was made up, but I mustered the strength to argue.

'Nah, mate. You're too young. That ain't happening.'

'I'm doing it.'

Soon, I was with Al's mum, Patsy, trying to persuade her to talk him out of it, trying to say that he had too much life in front of him, that I couldn't see him do this. She was as adamant as Al. His mind was made up. We ran the tests and he was a perfect match. They did find a spot on his liver that could jeopardise everything but it turned out to be from the protein shakes Al was taking (he loves the gym), and after a month off them, the spot was gone and we were good to go.

It was 2017, two years after I had discovered my illness. I remember the evening we headed off to the hospital. Unlike the night before Manchester United's Champions League final, sleep had not been a problem for me. Not that I wasn't nervous. I was stalling, though. I kept packing and unpacking my bag. 'Come on,' Shirley would say, 'we have to go.' I would unpack my bag again and make an excuse, saying I needed to make sure I had everything.

Eventually Shirley and the kids got me in the car. We were at the hospital, shown to our rooms. The doctors ran through the procedure: Alex will go down first, they'll take out his kidney, bring him up, take me down, do what they have to do, get the kidney working inside me, bring me up and see how my body takes it. Sounded simple enough!

And then it was just me and Al. His room was down the corridor and we sat together in comfortable silence. A knowing look was all it took to tell him how grateful I was. A smile back was all I needed to know he was determined to help.

'Do we really need to do this?' I kept asking the doctors. 'Can't you give me another week? I'll get better.' Questions met with silence.

They had let me go as far as they could. By now my kidney was down to 7 per cent of its usual capacity. It was time to get rid of it. I was scared. Not for me, but for the kids. I was stepping into my last-chance saloon. If this didn't work, that might be it, and I was scared for them.

It was a day of reckoning, I guess. Al was helping me have a chance at some sort of normal life. If it didn't work, I would have no life, and while I sat upstairs knowing my nephew was down there, giving up his kidney for that, I was overwhelmed with love and respect. And then it was my turn.

Shirley was great. She walked me down, but I was overcome with emotion. I broke down in tears. It wasn't fear for what was about to happen under a surgeon's scalpel. No, the tears that ran down my cheeks were for my family. I knew how serious this was now. Soon, with the tears still on my face and doctors making polite conversation, the anaesthetist was getting to work, and I was out.

I woke up desperate for a pee. I was groggy as hell, but that's what I remember. There was a voice. A woman's voice. 'Mr Cole, it's OK, just wee.'

What? I was thinking, 'I can't, you're a woman. I can't pee in front of a woman.' I was so desperate, though.

'It's OK,' she kept saying.

My morals must have subsided and I must have had that pee, but I can't remember how. I was in and out of consciousness. I could hear people talking. Eventually I could tell I was up in my room, my family around me, in and out. So groggy. Tubes everywhere. I could tell the room was a happy one. They were buzzing. 'It went so well,' I could hear the doctors saying. 'It was a great kidney,' they said. 'Really big, we had to make a bit more room in there.'

Alexander. As my thoughts became more coherent, they were all about my nephew. How is he? Apparently he was doing well and when I was finally allowed to get up, I would make my way to his room to check on him. Everything hurt. Everything was swollen. I was peeing into a bag that I was carrying around. It was so painful, but I wanted to know Alex was completely OK.

The thing is, he wasn't. It was clear that my nephew was in a lot of pain. He couldn't go to the toilet, and to see him in so much pain was the hardest thing. I was on at the doctors every day, pestering them to make him better, so much so I began to forget about my own discomfort.

It was a discomfort that my old captain Roy Keane clearly had no time for when he came to visit. Rather than bringing grapes or magazines, Skip brought his sense of humour. And despite being told by the nurses not to make me laugh, he sat by my bed, telling me old jokes, reminiscing about funny old times, making me laugh so much I feared for my stitches.

When Skip left, belly aches aside, I was on a high. For my old captain to take the time to see me meant so much. People have their views about Roy, but so much of public opinion is based purely on what people see on the surface. Skip is a class act and his being there at my bedside reminded me of that.

My high at his visit was matched by a trip to the loo, where for the first time in two years I stood and had a comfortable pee. What a fantastic feeling! After two years of very rarely peeing, that horrible feeling that my bladder was never really emptied, that had gone. Oh my God, it was pure joy. But, as happy as these things made me, there was still anxiety about Alex. Al's pain wouldn't go away, and no matter how good I was starting to feel, the thought of him struggling was eating me up. So much so that when the doctors said I could go home, I didn't want to leave him alone.

The doctors wanted me on my feet at home, though. I had to come in every day, but I was home, where I could rest without people checking me every five minutes. It should have been so sweet. But in my room, I broke down. Al was still in there. I prayed. I prayed, asking for Al to be up and out of there. I would go back to how I was before the operation if it meant he got better. This guy had put himself through all this, just to make me better. I couldn't get my head around what was happening. I was at home, hopefully on the mend, and the young man who had made that possible was doubled up in pain on a hospital bed. How can that be right?

After tests, the doctors discovered that Al had trapped gas, which was causing all the pain and his continued inability to go to the toilet. It might have been dangerous, but after a minor operation, the problem was solved. I would visit him every day and I think he knows just how grateful I am to him. The best moment was seeing Al walk tall out of that hospital. I had my nephew back. Patsy had her son back. Today he is fine. In fact, he was back in the gym a month or so later. A bit more tired than before, but he lives a normal and healthy life.

For me, life after the transplant was far from normal. I had had all that conflict with my medication, the side effects that they brought on, the depression and the suicidal thoughts that my situation had helped cause, and now my marriage was going to face challenges that no medication could solve.

Shirley could be so supportive, but there were times when she would say things, things so venomous that I didn't recognise her. On top of those rows I would have with my pills, I was constantly fighting my wife. Shirley was fighting me to go her way. She would read up on things and then her opinion was gospel. When I made it clear I was going to do things my way, or that I disagreed, she would take it as a knock against her, and become more and more disgruntled with me for ignoring her feelings. Day after day, more and more distant from each other.

We were back to where we had been when Faith wasn't well. Two people and an illness. This time, though, it was *my* illness, and while Shirley felt she knew what I was going through because she had nursed our daughter, she didn't, and how I dealt with it was not up for discussion.

'Embrace it,' she said. 'Embrace your new lease of life.'

That had me reeling. Are you mad? Transplant is not a cure; that's what so many people fail to realise. My new kidney gave me a chance of a life, a chance to get to tomorrow; it gave me a standard of life that gets me through the day. But I was mourning my previous healthy, active life, and Shirley couldn't get that.

She also called me selfish, suggesting that I had somehow put myself first through all this. That hurt so much. In that week after the transplant, with wires and tubes protruding out of me, all I had thought about was my family. I had a lawyer in to sort out my will, and with Devante turning down a contract from Manchester City as he wanted to play, my sole thought was that I had to get him a club. It must have looked odd to nurses as they fussed around me while I took meetings with football agents, desperate to get him a club, thinking if I don't get out of here I want to rest in peace, knowing my son had got a football club.

The relationship was struggling more and more every day. I would explain how I was feeling – usually very low – and I would get an answer from somewhere else. I didn't have the strength. I was angry that this had happened to us. I was tired of being tired, and in those first few months, when my body was most likely to reject the new organ, I was scared.

Early winter 2017 and things were at their worst. I was lower than I had ever been. Angry at my illness, hating my medication, depressed, suicidal even. I needed support, and there was none. I was getting the medical help I needed – pills, tests, all of that was sorted – but mentally I was adrift.

'I can't do this any more,' I said to Shirley that November. 'This thing is killing me. I'm not sure I can go through it any more.'

Shirley was despondent. Unable to help, unable to

muster any love that she might have once had for me. 'I can't do this any more either,' she said. I didn't know what she meant. 'This marriage is over.'

At first, I thought it was a flippant, angry comment. Something couples say to each other at the worst of times, but it soon dawned on me that these were very much the worst of times. For a while we lived a kind of half marriage, until end of 2018, when I got an email from Shirley's new lawyers with attached divorce papers. It made me laugh that the law firm was the same used by a couple of wives of certain team-mates I had played with. I guess there is money to be made in football heartbreak! At my lowest, there it was. My marriage was shattering right in front of my tired eyes. We would go on living with each other for a bit, but the damage was done.

Christmas 2017 was especially bad. I wanted to have a quiet one. I am not a Christmas man, never have been, but all I wanted was for my kids to be happy and I hoped with my low mood and my failing marriage, a quiet but cosy festive period would be best for everyone. I booked a local restaurant where we could all dine, but Shirley wasn't having it.

She wanted to have her family up from London, something we had often done, but why this year? I wanted peace and quiet. She had decided, though, and I started to go against her. If her family are coming, I said, then I will invite my family too.

Their fractious relationship with my wife meant they never came for Christmas, but with me now at constant loggerheads with Shirley and the marriage over, why shouldn't they? It was a typical family row about Christmas, but we were no longer a typical family.

So there it was. Twenty-seven years together. Ups and downs. Beautiful children, good times, horrific times and ultimately a relationship that was forever broken. I was at my lowest, but this wasn't about my illness, or how I was coping. Shirley had resented me for eight years, for how she felt I had let her down the week Faith was in hospital and the way I coped with that nightmare in our life. It was then and there that she had downed tools on our marriage. Nearly three decades had passed since I, a keen young footballer, had met her, but now it was over.

I was fighting my illness, so maybe it was best to stop fighting my wife. She had her resentment towards me and was no longer able to go through my illness with me. In September 2018, Shirley and Faith moved out. I was alone with my pills! There are good days and there are bad days. Some days I look at all my medication and we have an argument. 'I'm not inter-ested, not today,' I think, but then they stare back at me. I know I have to take them, and so I do. After all, another day lies ahead.

15

ANOTHER DAY

In the summer of 2019, I took myself and a mate to the All England Lawn Tennis and Croquet Club in Wimbledon to watch a bit of tennis. A lovely day out, made even better by a bit of banter. I'd been introduced to Jamie Delgado, Andy Murray's coach, through a mutual friend, and when he heard I was coming along, Jamie got in touch and said that Andy wanted to meet me.

Things like that seem strange to me. Andy Murray wants to meet me? Why? It turns out that Andy is a massive football fan, and with his coach being a Manchester United fan, he was keen to meet and laugh at my old club's current predicaments. 'Who does he support?' I asked Jamie.

'Arsenal.'

'Oh, bring it on.'

I met Andy and we had a real laugh. He had a go at United, I had a good go at Arsenal. Just like old times. Andy was great. The stick went back and forth and he even introduced me to the Williams sisters. Both Serena and Venus were equally as keen to talk football, saying they love to watch 'soccer' on the television at home and had enjoyed their country's recent win in the women's World Cup.

As I stood there, talking and laughing with such sporting elite, I wore an inner grin. My football career had given me so much and taken me to so many places, and now, retired, here I was rubbing shoulders with tennis royalty in the plushest of settings. Andrew, I thought to myself, 'you might have cracked it.'

There have been a few times I've thought that. Lining up to play in the Maracanã in Rio was one occasion; meeting a hero, Sócrates, in 2010 at the World Cup in South Africa was another. Standing in a tunnel preparing to face Brazil's Ronaldo. All split-second moments when I could think about where I'd come from, and where I had got myself.

I often think back to a day trip us boys had while at Lilleshall. The National School took us to a local prison (perhaps wanting to show some of us a worst-case scenario) and in there I recognised an inmate. He was one of my elders back home, one of those I would play football with, and he came over and said hello. We had a chat and when I rejoined my group, all the boys were shocked. 'You know that lad?' they asked. They couldn't quite believe I knew someone who was in prison. That made me laugh because I knew a few and was fully aware that without football and my talent for it, I could well have been in there myself.

I was lucky. I had been looked out for and I had made my way in the game, but I could never forget where I came from. The word 'journey' is overused, but I will always cherish the start of mine. That's why the end of my marriage upset me, as I felt that Shirley was forgetting our past.

When we met, we were teenagers. I had never ever wanted to get married – as a perhaps cynical young man with foresight, I dreaded the idea of a messy divorce – but we had a son and started a family as husband and wife.

Shirley was part of my journey. With me every step of the way. I knocked my pipe out working to get us a life neither of us could have even dreamt of. Her support, her brilliance as a mum, of course it was vital to our life, but then, with me suffering an illness and struggling with how to cope with new life-changing circumstances, all that disappeared and our life together was broken down into pounds, pence and bitterness.

I'm not sure if my split from Shirley left me heart-broken. It's strange to spend twenty-seven years together but not know the person you are ending that relation-ship with. I know I could have done things differently, and I apologise for my part in the end of our marriage, but moving forward, it saddens me that where we came from has been forgotten, the hard work has been forgotten, and now talk is only of perceived entitlement.

When Shirley declared that the marriage was over in

2017, I didn't know what to expect or what to feel. Nearly thirty years together, two wonderful children, but now it was over. It was hard. Very hard. Shirley's behaviour during what became a very difficult time was what I considered hugely unreasonable, crunching our decades together into mere pounds and pence.

There was also my daughter's illness, and my health; it was all on top. And then came the global Covid-19 pandemic. With my illness, I was instructed to lock down. Properly lock down. It meant I was alone in my rented flat, only opening the door to pick up groceries left by kind friends. I was in a bad way. I had many thoughts, my mind for the majority of the time my only companion, pondering on my career and, yes, the many mistakes I'd made. But it also dawned on me that I was blessed with a sense of pride, thinking about the many things I achieved in the game and the many friends I have made along the way. Friends, real friends, they are more valuable than any wealth a man can acquire through his life, and I'm not sure I would be here without them. Thank God for FaceTime chats with my children, my loving family and those friends, because otherwise I fear everything might have overwhelmed me.

It was a hard time. After my career ended and during my illness, I was involved in a fraud case. I can't talk too much about it because, as I write, the case is ongoing, but it was a classic case of former footballers being given sickeningly wrong business advice and falling victim to crime.

It is a scary stat that around 50 per cent of sports professionals go bankrupt after retirement. I and a few other ex-pros have come together and started an organisation called Phoenix Sport & Media Group, designed to assist both former and current athletes with their finances, helping to create employment opportunities for players after football, and by using a security and investigations company overseen by skilled ex-policemen and military operatives, we are there for sports stars who might otherwise fall foul of what is essentially crime. It's a great new project and, for me personally, it's now so uplifting that I am able to take the most difficult experiences in my life and try to help others.

Since I retired from football, I've learnt a lot about people and about myself, but I will move forward, and I will focus on the two most precious things to come out of my marriage, namely our children. Devante and Faith are so precious to me and it is now time for all of us to put things behind us, but I seriously don't think I could have without the support from the loved ones around me.

My sister Jackie, for example. The same sister who took me in when I moved to London as a raw teenager and became a second mum for me, she has never stopped looking out for me, especially in the last couple of years. Her son and my nephew Michael too, a constant companion; even my mates, brilliant blokes, able to talk things through with me, supporting me as I make my way through this new life.

What hasn't changed is my desire to work. I don't have idle hands and I have thrown myself into the work I do at Manchester United. Not only does it give me the chance to keep the smell of the game in my nostrils, but I have become fascinated by the business side of football, and marvel at the hard work that my colleagues at Old Trafford put in to get it right.

When I'm working with people (though nothing can replace the buzz a footballer gets in a dressing room) I love the camaraderie and the laughter that fills the working day. I may have once played on the pitch at Old Trafford, but today I am very much part of another team there, and despite my past, I am simply one of them. I remember Bryan Robson was with us one day, and a colleague called me 'Coley'. Robbo was surprised that they were so familiar with me, until I explained that that was just how it was.

My desire to work can cause me problems. My illness doesn't always share my fondness for graft and it lets me know in no uncertain terms. I hate it for that. I have a few football clinics for kids and on a recent visit to one in Portugal, I was coaching and buzzing off it.

I wanted to give more, so I did. I did a whole day, but the next morning I was empty. Totally empty.

I find that hard. Letting my illness win is not easy for me. There is no upside to being ill, and waking up unable to contribute to a day gives me the hump, but I am learning to listen to my body. Family and friends are more patient than me, and if I need to just sleep, they encourage it.

For me, a good day is waking up at 7 a.m., feeling energised and ready to get on with life. A bad day is being woken by my alarm at 9 a.m., the time I have to take my tablets. I look at them, they look back at me, they don't move and so I have to. I take them and then I may not get up until lunchtime, unable to function properly. Some days are a blur until I take my tablets again at 9 p.m. and go back to sleep for the night, hoping tomorrow will be different.

And often it is. One such occasion was when I went to the Houses of Parliament to lend a hand to a campaign run by the *Daily Mirror* to change the laws regarding organ donors. As a young, impetuous man I would probably have turned my nose up at the thought of being a donor, my body is a temple and all that, but my experiences have changed me, and while I was so lucky to have my nephew Alex, who was compatible and willing to give up his kidney for me, so many people are less fortunate and they have to rely on strangers for a chance of life.

Being part of that campaign and ultimately seeing the Organ Donation Bill (also known as Max and Keira's Law) passed and the laws changed so that from 2020 people will have to opt out of donating organs, rather than opting in, has been so rewarding. They say up to 700 lives a year will be saved and I was privileged to be any sort of help.

What was also a privilege was that by being part of the campaign I got to meet so many people and their families who were going through the same thing as me. What an eye-opener. As I talked to people, what surprised me was that all the fears and insecurities I had with my illness were so universal. I thought the way I was coping was unique. Self-doubting, self-loathing, it is so common amongst those who experience transplants, and to be able to talk that through with so many amazing people has been really helpful to me.

A common theme is self-repulsion. Organ failure can change so much in a person. I would stand in front of the mirror and feel only hate. I felt like a waste of space, no good to anyone. What was the point of me? I presumed that my life as a sportsman and the athleticism that life had given me had made me vain and that without the energy I once had as a footballer, how could I go on?

I thought these were feelings only someone like me might have, but then I met and talked to people from all walks of life and they shared their similar stories, making me realise that the way I was coping was common. I wasn't as mad as I thought!

I talked to members of families who have strived just to support their loved ones. These people understood that every day is different and you just don't know what mood someone might wake up in. The key is simply to support that mood in any way you can. It's so hard, but I realise that the resentment that started to dominate my marriage stemmed from that lack of communication and support.

I've set up the Andrew Cole Fund with Kidney Research UK, and we hope to raise vital money to help research into kidney disease, but also we want to support those going through not only the physical difficulties that come with the illness, but also the mental health issues that affect us all, living with a new normal every day.

I also got myself to Bristol to visit the research labs that specialise in kidney failure, and by having things broken down by specialists, my eyes have been opened further, and with knowledge of my illness, I have become more and more empowered against it. As my old skipper Roy Keane liked to say, 'Fail to prepare, prepare to fail.' It's OK, Skip, I'm preparing.

I'm not saying I've now sussed it. Life is a challenge and it always will be. It's just that I can now look at my illness in different ways. I can tackle it using different methods, when previously my only tactic was to be aggressive and attack it. I had approached football that way, but in time I realised that this ain't football.

A mate of mine summed it up when he said that I had always had only one tool in my box – a hammer. That made me laugh and he's right. A problem? I'll take my hammer to it. Conflict? I'll take my hammer to it. In time and by talking to people, I have been able to put the hammer down. Don't get me wrong, I still have it and it can still come out, but I'm learning to cope in other ways.

And what of the future? I used to daydream of a family living in a house with the white picket fence and grandkids everywhere. The family dynamic has changed, and the picket fence has come down, but I of course think about my future and my kids. They are and always will be at the forefront of my mind. As is the case for any children dealing with divorce, it hasn't been easy, but they are two incredible people, taking on their own challenges, and I couldn't be more proud of them.

Faith continues to inspire us all. My little angel has grown up into a remarkable young woman, coping with her own illness, writing a blog about her experiences, helping others with her wise words. She is off to university and refuses to become subservient to her illness. There are days she needs to just stay in her room (what teenager doesn't have those days?), and I get that better than anyone, but I'm constantly in awe as I watch her take on life with such spirit and grace.

Devante has had to watch both his sister and his dad fall ill, wondering if he might lose one or even both of us. It must have been so hard for him, but he has handled it all with quiet strength. It is the same way he has gone about his football career. It isn't easy, but Devante's love for the game shines through.

For me, it has been hard to watch at times. Football can be harsh and I have been upset on several occasions as clubs and their managers deal with young footballers as if dealing with cattle, but Devante's dedication to the game is incredible and he always conducts himself so well, even if I am losing my rag behind the scenes.

I've had a few run-ins with his clubs. I remember when Brian Marwood at Manchester City took a condescending tone with me when I argued Devante's case regarding a proposed move from City to Brentford. It was a loan deal leading to a permanent move, but Devante had absolutely no say in it. He could do brilliantly on loan, a bigger club could come in for him, but he would have to sign with Brentford. That's not right.

Brian took a tone I didn't care for and I had to remind him I was no longer the youth-team player who cleaned his boots at Arsenal in the late 1980s. I get that a lot.

Uwe Rösler was Devante's manager at Fleetwood Town and he couldn't help but be patronising. He made me laugh, and again I had to put him right, reminding him that I played at the highest level and the fact that he has become a manager doesn't make him better than anyone. I can sit down with Sir Alex Ferguson and talk about football. He will ask my opinion and I'll give it. If Sir Alex can talk to me without talking down to me, then so can Uwe Rösler.

I try not to be Devante's agent. He's his own man. On one occasion, when I was very ill, we fell out. The time I had been in a hospital bed, trying hard, maybe too hard, to get him a new contract was tricky for us all, but it got trickier when I got home and found out Paul Stretford had been contacted and agreed to help my son. With everything that had gone on with me and Paul, I felt a huge betrayal and made my feelings known. Devante and I are always ok, and we sorted it out but at the time, it put a strain on the family.

Devante takes it in his stride. As his father looking in, I find it strange to see him facing the same old prejudices that I can remember. Devante is a confident young man, but in football, even today, a confident young black player is labelled as having an attitude problem. I have to laugh when I hear him getting the same stuff I used to. A white footballer who argues his corner is confident, a black player with the same characteristics is a problem and needs taking down a peg or two. I went through all that, but now as a parent, I find it hard to accept and it angers me that, as we approach 2020, football still holds on to its old prejudices. Racism is society's problem, one that rears its ugly head in the game, but what can football do to combat it?

The ultimate cure comes outside the sport and in classrooms and households, where hate can be eroded, but organisations such as Kick It Out need to have more power. The odd weekend where players wear T-shirts during their warm-up isn't enough, and for all the good work it does, Kick It Out needs to seek out more power within the game and the outside world.

Devante has been on the end of racism at home and abroad. When he was starting out, he called me once after playing in Spain with Manchester City, clearly upset with the abuse that had come his way. That was hard. To hear how broken he was and not be able to assure him that this was just a one-off made me angry and worried for where we all are.

If anything, it seems that Devante's career will be even more blighted by racism than my own. The modern world seems to have given a more accepted platform to bigotry and hate, and with the outside world so divisive, football will only magnify it. That is a worry for me, as both a proud black man and the father of a young black footballer.

*

I have had a go at coaching and loved it. I worked with the strikers at Huddersfield with my old mate Lee Clark, and at Macclesfield and then Southend, with another old mate, Sol Campbell. I've dipped my toe in, but management isn't for me. For one, I don't quite know how I would handle someone like me, but I am also put off by the obstacles set in front of young black managers such as Sol.

Sol Campbell had a brilliant playing career. His experiences and his quality surely make him ideal management material. The job he did under incredibly difficult circumstances at both Macclesfield and Southend, where finances were more than tight, should have made him a hot property, but black managers don't seem to get the same opportunities. They say everyone starts on a level playing field, but I'm not having that. Sol's white peers are getting more chances to coach and manage and I just don't see anything like a level playing field.

There was a time when the English game embraced a couple of black managers: Jean Tigana and Ruud Gullit. Yes, they were black but they were seen as exotic. French and Dutch respectively. Brilliant players in stylish teams. It was as if football could see past the colour of their skin. English black players wanting to manage are left with the old prejudices that pioneering players in the 1970s and 1980s suffered. Namely, that they are luxuries, not hard workers, not deep thinkers, and therefore incapable of running a team. It's not right and it has to change.

Football can anger me but I remain a huge fan. It is the sport I have always loved and always will love. What I would like to see the game do is harness the power that it has. Football brings people together and I would like to see governing bodies take their eyes away from their balance sheets and try to utilise the very real good the game can bring to a troubled world. I'll watch on with interest.

I somehow made it in the game and managed to achieve more than I could have dreamt of, and more than I am perhaps comfortable acknowledging. Former team-mates remind me to pat myself on the back sometimes, and maybe they're right.

My illness might be the thing that finishes me, but I won't go without a right good battle. Recently, I spoke with Ian Wright and said just that. When I suggested the mere possibility that one day the illness might win, he wasn't having it. 'Coley,' he said, 'you have fought your whole life and most of those battles you have won. You are not going to lose this one. No chance.' Typical Wrighty.

Time will tell if he's right, but I know I have the tools to take it on. The hammer is still there and will be used now and then, but I have family, I have support, and I have love. My sister recently asked me if I ever think I could meet someone new. She received an emphatic no. I am closed off to all that. My sister says that one day I will change my mind, and maybe she is right. For now, I am learning to love myself again, learning to be less toxic about myself. Once that is sorted, you never know.

Today I can get close to the hope that transplants give people. In August 2019, I attended the World Transplant Games in Newcastle. It was the most inspiring of events. Competitors from all over the world, all having gone through organ transplants, and all pushing themselves to the very limit. The GB football team had me in tears. I was there to support them, but they showed me so much love back, and that shared love among people who have gone through this is something that spurs me on, even on the hardest of days.

If I'm not crying, you'll find me laughing. I mentioned earlier that, despite that public perception of me as serious and deep-thinking, there is nothing I like better than being with old mates, and basically ripping each other to bits with our humour. All footballers will tell you they miss the dressing room, the never-ending digs and laughs, and I do too, but I am lucky that even when I was a footballer, I had a set of mates detached from my day job. Yes, they all love football and they would talk about it, but when we went on our annual holidays (we still go) I could just be 'Coley', their mate, the bloke they would take the mickey out of, and the bloke who would readily take the mickey out of them. I cherish them all.

The people I have around me now are more than enough. Today, my dad and I are so close. We talk loads – not about football, as he still just doesn't get it – and I love him so much. In so many ways he is my hero, a man who came to England from his beautiful Caribbean home, took all sorts of abuse quietly and with dignity, and worked hard to give his family opportunities. Mum too. I am a mummy's boy and can't thank her enough for all the love and support she continues to give me. Mum and Pops are my king and queen.

So that's my story. An ambitious and angry young footballer who made his way from Nottingham to London to find his fortune. I've taken the roads from Bristol to Newcastle, to Manchester and beyond, and you know what, I did all right.

There were doubters along the way, but they made me stronger and I can only genuinely thank all of my coaches, even those who doubted me, for they added fuel to my already bright fire. There are no grudges. There is no time for all that. Instead, I look back with pride and look forward with hope. Tomorrow really is another day.

ACKNOWLEDGEMENTS

I'd like to thank a number of people for the help they gave me in putting this book together. First of all, Roddy Bloomfield, Huw Armstrong and their fantastic team at Hodder. Thank you all for your support and efforts.

Leo Moynihan has been brilliant to work with. Leo has spent so much of the last eight months with me, and I thank him not only for getting my thoughts and memories down so well on these pages, but also for sharing so many laughs . . . and tears. Yes, I saw them! I'd also like to thank literary agent David Luxton for his never-ending enthusiasm for the book. Thanks to Sir Alex Ferguson for his Foreword. The gaffer didn't always get thanks from me, but he remains the greatest football man I ever worked with and I thank him for his kind words.

I'd also like to thank Craig Short, Michael Thomas, Brian Deane, Rod Wallace, Paul Williams, Tommy Johnson, Craig Morris and Dave Matthews; and a special mention to Carly Barnes and Ben Rees for their tireless and constant support.

I want to say thank you to all my team-mates. It's been a blast. Some supported me more than others, but life is too short to hold grudges and I have loved sharing my career with you all. Also thanks to all my old managers, coaches and backroom staff. Without so many people behind the scenes, us footballers are nothing.

My biggest thanks, though, must go to my family and friends. To my mum and my pops. Without you there would have been no football career. My brother Desmond and my six sisters, Patricia, Jacqueline, Joy, Marva, Lorraine and Sybil, and my brother-in-law, Clifton. Thank you all for your never-ending love. My nieces and my nephews, Michael, Charlene, Kamar, thank you for your support and jokes. And Alexander, my brave nephew, who gave me the opportunity to continue living a decent life, I cannot thank you enough.

Andrew Cole,
September 2020

PHOTOGRAPHIC ACKNOWLEDGEMENTS

The author and publisher would like to thank the following for permission to reproduce photographs:

Section One
Mark Leech/Getty Images, Paul Marriott/EMPICS Sport, Graham Chadwick/EMPICS Sport, Shaun Botterill/Getty Images, David Kendall/ PA Archive/PA Images, Anton Want/ALLSPORT/Getty Images, Shaun Botterill /Allsport/Getty Images, Aubrey Washington/EMPICS Sport, Phil Noble/PA Archive/PA Images, Michael Steele/EMPICS Sport, Ben Radford /Allsport/Getty Images, Neal Simpson/EMPICS Sport, Shaun Botterill / Allsport/ Getty Images, Michael Steele/EMPICS Sport, Popperfoto via Getty Images, Owen Humphreys/PA Archive/PA Images, Michael Steele/ EMPICS Sport, www.imago-images.de/Imago/PA Images

Section Two
Matthew Ashton/EMPICS Sport, Martin Rickett/PA Archive/PA Images, Matthew Ashton/EMPICS Sport, David Ashdown/Getty Images, Gareth Copley/PA Archive/PA Images, Alex Livesey/Getty Images, John Walton/ EMPICS Sport, Neal Simpson/EMPICS Sport, Nick Potts/PA Archive/PA Images, Allsport UK/Getty Images, John Stillwell/PA Archive/PA Images, Steve Mitchell/EMPICS Sport, John Stillwell/PA Archive/PA Images

All other photographs are from private collections.

Every reasonable effort has been made to trace the copyright holders, but if there are any errors or omissions, Hodder & Stoughton will be pleased to insert the appropriate acknowledgements in any subsequent printings or editions.

INDEX

INDEX